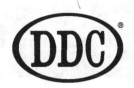

Internet in an Hour

Health & Medical Resources

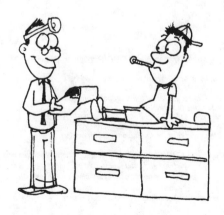

Acknowledgments

Managing Editor

Jennifer Frew

Technical and English Editors

David Lott
Monique Peterson

Design and Layout

Midori Nakamura
Shu Chen
Maria Kardasheva
Paul Wray

Cover Design and Layout

Amy Capuano

Illustrations

Ryan Sather

Contributing Authors

Jennifer Frew
David Lott
Monique Peterson

Editorial Assistant

Emily Hay

Copyright© 1999 by DDC Publishing, Inc.
Published by DDC Publishing, Inc.

ISBN: 1-56243-713-5
Cat. No. HR10
DDC Publishing, Inc. Printing:
10   9   8   7   6   5   4   3   2   1
Printed in the United States of America.

IMPORTANT NOTE
TO READERS

The information contained in this book and on the Web sites featured herein is not intended as a substitute for consulting with a doctor, health care provider, or other medical professional. The material published in this book is for general educational purposes only. The publisher and authors do not take responsibility for the information, advice, or opinions found at any of the Web sites or links featured in this book. Persons accessing the Web sites featured in this book assume full responsibility for the use of the material found at those sites. Always consult a doctor pertaining to all matters of your physical and mental health.

Contents

WEB RESOURCES

Contents

Introduction

This Book Is Designed for You ..

if you are interested in exploring the wealth of medical information on the World Wide Web. You'll learn how to get online and get the search results you want quickly. Find answers to all your questions, learn about the latest in medical research, and locate community support near you.

The book is divided into two sections: Basics and Web Resources.

Basics

In Internet Basics, you'll learn how to:

- Use Netscape Navigator to browse the World Wide Web.
- Use Internet Explorer to browse the World Wide Web.
- Access the Internet using America Online.
- Send and receive e-mail with Netscape Messenger, Microsoft Outlook Express, and America Online.
- Find information on the Web with search engines.

Web Resources

In the Web Resources section, you'll discover many of the best health and medical resources that the Web has to offer. Whether you are looking for quick relief for an earache or you want to read up on the latest research on diabetes, this book shows you where to find answers. Keep in mind, however, as you surf these sites that although consulting the Web can be an excellent way to access resources, it is by no means a substitute for consulting a qualified physician.

What Do I Need to Use This Book?

This book assumes that you have some general knowledge and experience with computers and that you already know how to perform the following tasks:

- Use a mouse (double-click, etc.).
- Make your way around Microsoft Windows 95.
- Install and run programs.

If you are completely new to computers, as well as to the World Wide Web, you may want to refer to DDC's *Learning Microsoft Windows 95* or *Learning the Internet.*

This book also assumes that you have an Internet connection and access to browser applications such as Microsoft Internet Explorer 4.0, Netscape Navigator 4.0, or America Online.

✔ *If you do not currently have these applications, contact your Internet Service Provider for instructions on how to download them. You can also use other browsers or previous versions such as Explorer 3.0 and Navigator 3.0 to browse the Web.*

✔ *This book does not cover how to get connected to the Internet.*

Please read over the following list of "must haves" to ensure that you are ready to be connected to the Internet:

- A computer (with a recommended minimum of 16 MB of RAM) and a modem port.
- A modem (with a recommended minimum speed of 14.4 kbps, and a suggested speed of 28.8 kbps) that is connected to an analog phone line (assuming you are not using a direct Internet connection through a school, corporation, etc.).
- Established access to the Internet through an online service, independent Internet Service Provider, etc.
- A great deal of patience. The Internet is a fun and exciting place, but getting connected can be frustrating at times. Expect to run into occasional glitches, get disconnected from time to time, or experience sporadic difficulty in viewing certain Web pages and features. The more up-to-date your equipment and software are, however, the less difficulty you will probably experience.

Internet Cautions

ACCURACY:

- Be careful not to believe everything on the Internet. Almost anyone can publish information on the Internet, and since there is no Internet editor or monitor, some information may be false. All information found on the World Wide Web should be checked for accuracy through additional reputable sources.

SECURITY:

- When sending information over the Internet, be prepared to let the world have access to it. Computer hackers can find ways to access anything that you send to anyone over the Internet, including e-mail. Be cautious when sending confidential information to anyone.

VIRUSES:

- These small, usually destructive computer programs hide inside of innocent-looking programs. Once a virus is executed, it attaches itself to other programs. When triggered, often by the occurrence of a date or time on the computer's internal clock/calendar, it can execute functions that are merely annoying (such as displaying a message on your screen) or ones that do more serious damage (such as corrupting your files or reformatting your hard drive).

BASICS

Netscape Navigator: 1

◆ About Netscape Navigator
◆ Start Netscape Navigator ◆ The Netscape Screen
◆ Exit Netscape Navigator

About Netscape Navigator

- This chapter focuses on Netscape Navigator 4.0, the Internet browser component of Netscape Communicator. Netscape Messenger, the e-mail component, is covered in Chapters 4-6.

Start Netscape Navigator

1. Click the Start button 🔳 Start .
2. Click Programs, Netscape Communicator, Netscape Navigator.
   OR

   If you have a shortcut to Netscape Communicator 📷 on your desktop, double-click it to start Netscape Navigator.

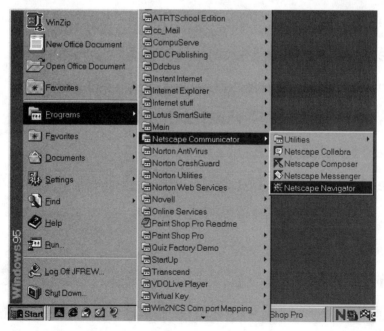

✔ *The first time you start Netscape Communicator, the New Profile Setup dialog box appears. Enter e-mail and service provider information in the dialog boxes that appear. If you do not know the information, you can leave it blank until you are ready to fill it in. See the sections on Netscape Messenger in this book for more information.*

The Netscape Screen

■ The Netscape Navigator screen contains features that help you explore the Internet. Some of these features are constant and some change depending on the task attempted or completed.

Title bar

Displays the name of the program (Netscape) and the current Web page (Welcome to Netscape).

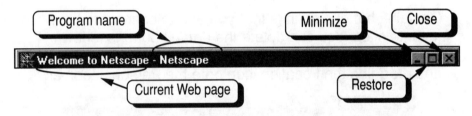

Menu bar

Displays drop-down lists of Netscape commands.

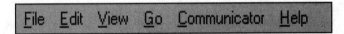

Navigation toolbar

Contains buttons for online activity. The name and icon on each button identify the command.

✔ *If the toolbar buttons are not visible, open the View menu and click Show Navigation Toolbar.*

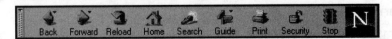

Location toolbar

The electronic address of the current Web page displays in the Location field. You can also type the Web page address, called a Uniform Resource Locator (URL), in the Location field and press Enter to access it.

✔ *If the Location toolbar is not visible, open the View menu and click Show Location Toolbar.*

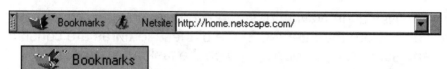

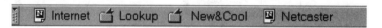

The Bookmarks QuickFile button is also on the Location toolbar. Click to view a list of sites that you have bookmarked for quick access. (For more on Bookmarks, see page 13.)

Personal toolbar

Contains buttons or links that you add to connect to your favorite sites. You can delete the default buttons (shown below) and add your own by displaying the desired Web site and dragging the Location icon onto the Personal toolbar.

Netscape's status indicator

Netscape's icon pulses when Netscape is processing a command. Click to return to Netscape's home page.

Status bar

When a Web page is opening, the Status bar indicates the downloading progress and the security level of the page being loaded. When you place the cursor over a hyperlink, the Status bar displays the URL of the link.

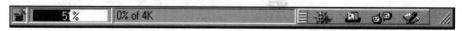

Component toolbar

The buttons on this toolbar link to other Netscape components: Navigator, Messenger Mailbox, Collabra Discussions, and Page Composer.

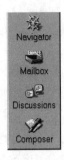

Exit Netscape Navigator

■ Exiting Netscape Navigator and disconnecting from your Internet Service Provider (ISP) are two separate steps. You can disconnect from your service provider and still have Netscape Navigator open. You can also disconnect from Navigator and still have your ISP open.

■ You may want to disconnect from your ISP and keep Netscape open to:

- Read information obtained from the Web

- Access information stored on your hard disk using Netscape

- Compose e-mail to send later

■ If you don't disconnect from your ISP and you pay an hourly rate, you will continue incurring charges.

✔ *You can disconnect from your ISP and still view Web information accessed during the current session by using the Back and Forward toolbar buttons. Your computer stores the visited sites in its memory.*

Netscape Navigator: 2

◆ The Navigation Toolbar
◆ Open World Wide Web Sites

The Navigation Toolbar

- The Netscape Navigation toolbar displays buttons for Netscape's most commonly used commands. Note that each button contains an icon and a word describing the button's function. Choosing any of these buttons activates the indicated task immediately.

- If the Navigation toolbar is not visible, select Show Navigation Toolbar from the View menu.

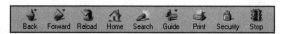

 Moves back through pages previously displayed. Back is available only if you have moved around among Web pages in the current Navigator session; otherwise, it is dimmed.

 Moves forward through pages previously displayed. Forward is available only if you have used the Back button; otherwise, it is dimmed.

 Reloads the currently displayed Web page. Use this button if the current page is taking too long to display or to update the current page with any changes that may have occurred since the page was downloaded.

 Displays the home page.

 Displays Netscape's Net Search Page. You can select one of several search tools from this page.

 Displays a menu with helpful links to Internet sites that contain search tools and services.

Prints the displayed page, topic, or article.

 Displays security information for the displayed Web page as well as information on Netscape security features.

 Stops the loading of a Web page.

Open World Wide Web Sites

- There are several ways to access a Web site. If you know the site's address, you can enter the correct Web address (URL) on the Location field on the Location toolbar.

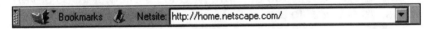

- If the address you are entering is the address of a site you have visited recently or that you have bookmarked (see page 13 for more information on Bookmarks), you will notice as you begin to type the address that Netscape attempts to complete it for you. If the address that Netscape suggests is the one you want, press Enter.

- If the address that Netscape suggests is not correct, keep typing to complete the desired address and then press Enter. Or, you can click the down arrow next to the Location field to view a list of other possible matches, select an address, and press Enter.

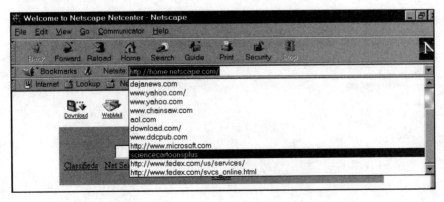

- There are a couple of shortcuts for entering URL addresses. One shortcut involves omitting the **http://www.** prefix from the Web address. Netscape assumes the **http://** protocol and the **www** that indicates that the site is located on the Web.

- If you are trying to connect to a company Web site, entering the company name is generally sufficient. Netscape assumes the **.com** suffix. For example, entering **ddcpublishing** on the location line and pressing Enter would reach the **http://www.ddcpub.com** address.

  ✔ *Don't be discouraged if you can't connect to the World Wide Web site immediately. The site may be offline temporarily. The site may also be very busy with other users trying to access it. Be sure the URL is typed accurately. Occasionally, it takes several tries to connect to a site.*

Netscape Navigator: 3

History List

- While you move back and forth among Web sites, Netscape automatically records each of these site locations in a History list, which is temporarily stored on your computer.

- You can use the History list to track or view sites that you have recently visited. The History list is an easy way to see the path you followed to get to a particular Web page.

- To view the History list, click History on the Communicator menu, or press Ctrl+H. To link to a site shown in the History list, double-click on it.

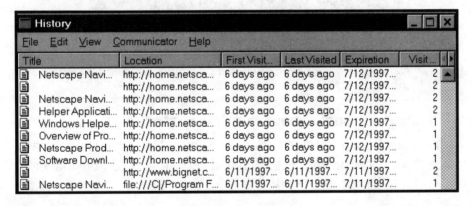

Bookmarks

- A Bookmark is a placeholder containing the title and URL of a Web page that, when selected, links directly to that page. If you find a Web site that you like and want to revisit, you can create a Bookmark to record its location. (See **Add Bookmarks** on the following page.)

- The Netscape Bookmark feature maintains permanent records of the Web sites in your Bookmark files so that you can return to them easily.

- You can view the Bookmarks menu by selecting <u>B</u>ookmarks from the <u>C</u>ommunicator menu or by clicking on the Bookmarks QuickFile button 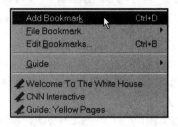 on the Location toolbar. The drop-down menu shown below appears.

Add Bookmarks

To add a Bookmark from an open Web page:

- Display the Web page to add, go to <u>B</u>ookmarks on the <u>C</u>ommunicator menu and click Add Bookmar<u>k</u>.

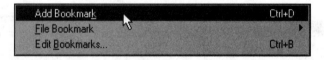

✔ *Netscape does not confirm that a bookmark has been added to the file.*

To create a Bookmark from the History list:

1. Click <u>C</u>ommunicator, <u>H</u>istory and select the listing to bookmark.
2. Right-click on your selection and choose Add To Bookmar<u>k</u>s from the pop-up menu.

Delete Bookmarks

- Bookmarks may be deleted at anytime. For example, you may wish to delete a Bookmark if a Web site no longer exists or is no longer of interest to you.

To delete a Bookmark:

1. Click <u>C</u>ommunicator.
2. Click <u>B</u>ookmarks.
3. Click Edit <u>B</u>ookmarks.

4. In the Bookmarks window, select the Bookmark you want to delete by clicking on it from the Bookmark list.

5. Press the Delete key.

OR

Right-click on the Bookmark and select <u>D</u>elete Bookmark from the pop-up menu as shown in the following illustration.

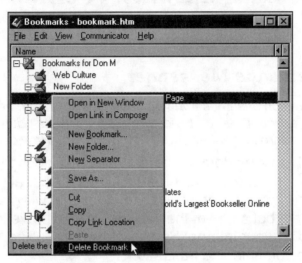

Print Web Pages

- You can print all information you find on the Internet.

To print a Web page:

✔ *Only displayed pages can be printed.*

1. Click the Print button [Print] on the Navigation toolbar.

OR

Click <u>F</u>ile, <u>P</u>rint.

2. In the Print dialog box that displays, select the desired print options and click [OK].

- In most cases, the Web page will be printed in the format shown in the Web page display.

Netscape Messenger: 4

◆ Start Netscape Messenger
◆ Configure Netscape Messenger
◆ The Message List Window ◆ Get New Mail
◆ Read Messages ◆ Delete a Message
◆ Print Messages

Start Netscape Messenger

✔ *This section assumes that you have already set up an e-mail account with a service provider. If you do not have an e-mail address, contact your Internet Service Provider.*

■ Establishing a modem connection and configuring your computer to send and receive mail can be frustrating. Don't be discouraged. What follows are steps that will get you connected, but some of the information may have to be supplied by your Internet Service Provider. Calling for help will save you time and frustration.

- Click the Mailbox icon ▦ ▦ on the Component bar from the Navigator window.

OR

Start Netscape Messenger from the Netscape Communicator submenu on the Start, <u>P</u>rograms menu.

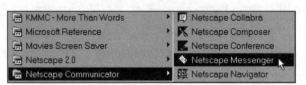

📰 KMMC - More Than Words ▸	🗐 Netscape Collabra
📰 Microsoft Reference ▸	🗡 Netscape Composer
📰 Movies Screen Saver ▸	📕 Netscape Conference
📰 Netscape 2.0 ▸	◈ Netscape Messenger
📰 Netscape Communicator ▸	🕮 Netscape Navigator

Configure Netscape Messenger

- Using Netscape Messenger you can send, receive, save, and print e-mail messages and attachments. First, you must configure the program with your e-mail account information.

- You may have already filled in this information if you completed the New Profile Setup Wizard when you installed Netscape Communicator.

- If not, follow these steps to get connected. You can also use these steps to change your e-mail setting.

Step 1: Identity Settings

- From the Navigator or Messenger menu:

  1. Click Edit and select Preferences.

  2. Double-click the Mail & Groups Category to display the list and click Identity.

  3. Enter your name, e-mail address, and any optional information in the Identity dialog boxes.

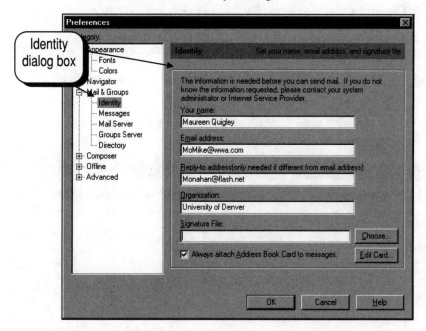

Step 2: Mail Server Preference Settings

- Completing this step will allow you to send and receive mail.

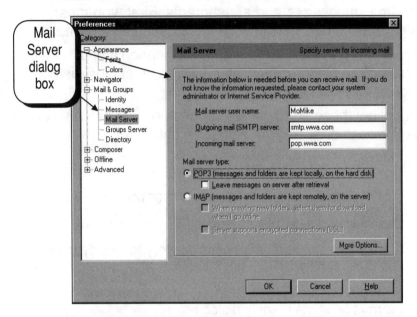

Mail Server dialog box

1. Click Mail Server from the Mail & Groups Category.

2. Enter your mail server user name. This is the part of your e-mail address that appears in front of the @ sign.

3. Enter your outgoing and incoming mail server address information.

   ✔ *Check with your ISP if you don't already have this information.*

4. Click [OK] to save and close the preference settings.

   ✔ *You should now be able to send and receive e-mail messages.*

The Message List Window

- After you launch Messenger, a message list window will open, displaying the contents of the e-mail Inbox folder. You can retrieve, read, forward, and reply to messages from this window.

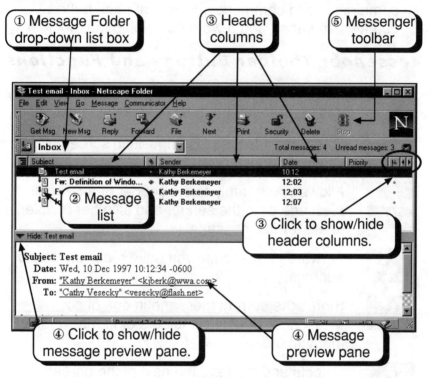

① Message Folder drop-down list box

③ Header columns

⑤ Messenger toolbar

② Message list

③ Click to show/hide header columns.

④ Click to show/hide message preview pane.

④ Message preview pane

- The message list window includes the following:

  ① The Message Folder drop-down list box displays the currently selected message folder. Click the down arrow to display a list of other message folders.

  ② The message list displays header information for each of the messages contained in the selected folder.

  ③ Header columns list the categories of information available for each message, such as subject, sender, and date.

④ The message preview pane displays the content of the message currently selected from the message list. You can show/hide the preview pane by clicking on the blue triangle icon in the bottom-left corner of the message list pane.

⑤ The Messenger toolbar displays buttons for activating commonly used commands. Note that each button contains an image and a word describing the function.

Messenger Toolbar Buttons and Functions

 Retrieves new mail from your Internet mail server and loads it into the Inbox message folder.

 Opens the Message Composition screen allowing you to compose new mail messages.

 Allows you to reply to the sender of an e-mail message or to the sender and all other recipients of the e-mail message.

 Forwards a message you have received to another address.

 Stores the current message in one of six Messenger default file folders or in a new folder that you create.

 Selects and displays the next of the unread messages in your Inbox.

 Prints the displayed message.

 Displays the security status of a message.

 Deletes the selected message. Deleted messages are moved to the Trash folder.

Get New Mail

- You must be connected to your ISP to access new e-mail messages.

To retrieve new messages:

1. Click the Get Msg button 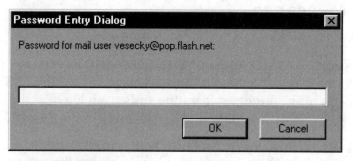 on the Messenger toolbar. (If you do not know your e-mail password, contact your ISP.)

2. If you have not instructed Netscape Messenger to save your password, you will have to enter it in the Password Entry dialog box that follows.

Password Entry Dialog

Password for mail user vesecky@pop.flash.net:

[OK   ] [Cancel   ]

3. Click [OK   ].

- The Getting New Messages box opens, displaying the status of your message retrieval.

Getting New Messages

Status: Connect: Host contacted, sending login information...

[Cancel]

- Once your new messages are retrieved, they are listed in the message list window. By default, Messenger stores new mail messages in the Inbox folder.

To save your Password permanently in Messenger:

1. Click Edit, Preferences.
2. Click on Mail Server under the Mail & Groups Category to select it.

   ✔ *If the Mail & Groups menu is not displayed, expand the list by clicking the + sign next to the Mail & Groups category.*

3. Click the More Options button [More Options...].
4. Select the Remember my mail password check box and click [OK] twice to save and exit Preferences.

Read Messages

- There are two ways to read messages:

  - You can read a message in the message preview pane located directly below the message list window. Single-click on a message from the message list and the contents of the message will appear in the preview pane.

    ✔ *If the message does not appear, the preview pane may be hidden. Click on the blue triangle icon at the bottom of the message list window to show the preview pane.*

    OR

    Double-click on the message from the message list to open it in its own window.

To close a message:

- Click File, Close.

  OR

  Click on the Close button (X) in the upper-right corner of the window.

To read the next unread message:

- Click the Next button [Next] on the Messenger toolbar.

  OR

  If you have reached the end of the current message, you can press the spacebar to proceed to the next unread message.

- Once you have read a message, it remains stored in the Inbox folder until you delete it or file it in another folder. (See **Delete a Message** below.)

  ✔ *You do not have to be online to read e-mail. You can reduce your online time by disconnecting from your ISP after retrieving your messages.*

  ✔ *Icons located to the left of message headers in the message list identify each message as either unread [icon] (retrieved during a previous Messenger session), new [icon] (and unread), or read [icon].*

Delete a Message

- There are two steps required to delete a message permanently. Deleting a message from the message list moves the message to the Trash folder. You must then delete it from the Trash folder to remove it permanently from your hard disk.

  1. To delete a message, click on the message to select it from the message list window.

  2. Click the Delete button [Delete] on the Messenger toolbar.

To delete messages from the Trash folder:

- Click Empty Trash Folder from the File menu to delete all items stored there.

  OR

  Delete the desired message by selecting it and pressing the Delete key.

✔ *To select more than one message to delete, hold the Ctrl button while you click each message to delete. Once all the desired messages are selected, press the Delete key.*

Print Messages

■ The message must first be open in order to print it.

1. Click the Print button [Print] on the Messenger toolbar.
2. In the Print dialog box that appears, select the desired print options and click [OK].

Netscape Messenger: 5

◆ New E-Mail Messages
◆ The Message Composition Toolbar
◆ Compose and Send Messages
◆ Reply to Mail ◆ Forward Mail
◆ Add Entries to the Personal Address Book
◆ Address a New Message Using the Personal
Address Book

New E-Mail Messages

- You can compose an e-mail message in Netscape Messenger on- or offline.

- After composing an e-mail message online, you have three choices:

  - send the message immediately

  - store the message in the Unsent Messages folder to be sent later (File, Send Later)

  - save the message in the Drafts folder to be finished and sent later (File, Save Draft)

- After composing a message offline (which frees up your phone line and also reduces any hourly ISP charges), store the message in your Unsent Messages folder until you are online and can send it.

The Message Composition Toolbar

- The toolbar in the Message Composition window has several features that are specific only to the message composition screen.

Message Composition Toolbar
Buttons and Functions

 Immediately sends current message.

 Used when replying to a message, the Quote feature allows you to include text from the original message.

 Select an address from the addresses stored in your personal Address Book to insert into address fields.

 By clicking the Attach button, you can send a file, a Web page, or your personal address card along with your e-mail message.

 Checks for spelling errors in the current message.

 Lets you save your message as a draft for later use.

 Sets the security status of a message.

 Stops the display of an HTML message or a message with an HTML attachment.

Compose and Send Messages

- There are four steps to composing and sending a basic e-mail message using Netscape Messenger:

Step 1: New Message

1. Click the New Message button 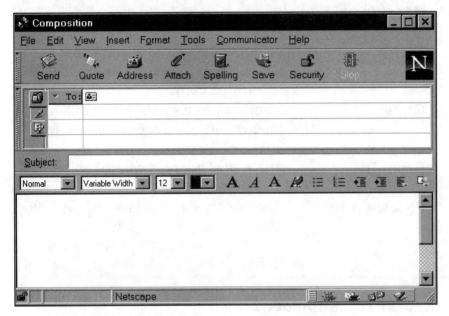 from the Messenger main screen.

    OR

    Press Ctrl+M.

    ✔ *The Message Composition window displays.*

2. In the Message Composition window, type the e-mail address(es) of the message recipient(s) in the To field.

    ✔ *If you are sending the message to multiple recipients, press Enter after typing each recipient's address to move to the next address line.*

    OR

    Click the Address button Address on the Message Composition toolbar and select an address to insert from the Address Book (see pages 27-29 for more information on using the Address Book).

- Click the To button ![To button] to display a drop-down menu of addressee options. Click on any of following options to enter the recipient information indicated:

To	The e-mail address of the person to whom the message is being sent.
CC (Carbon Copy)	The e-mail addresses of people who will receive copies of the message.
BCC (Blind Carbon Copy)	Same as CC, except these names will not appear anywhere in the message, so other recipients will not know that the person(s) listed in the BCC field received a copy.
Group	Names of Newsgroups that will receive this message (similar to Mail To).
Reply To	The e-mail address where replies should be sent.
Follow-up To	Another Newsgroup heading; used to identify Newsgroups to which comments should be posted (similar to Reply To).

Step 2: The Subject

- Click in the Subject field (or press Tab to move the cursor there) and type a banner for your message. This is the first thing the recipient will see announcing your e-mail message. The subject should be a few-word summation of your message.

Step 3: The Message

- Click to or Tab down to the blank composition area below the Subject field and type the body of your message.

To spell-check your e-mail message:

- Check the spelling of your message by clicking on the

  Spelling button [Spelling] on the Message Composition
  toolbar and respond to the dialog prompts that follow.

Step 4: Sending the Message

To send a message immediately:

- Click the Send button [Send] on the Message Composition
  toolbar.

To send a message later:

- Use these procedures to send message that you
  compose offline or that you wish to send later.

  - Click File, Send Later.

    OR

    Click File, Save Draft.

- Saving the message in the Drafts folder lets you finish
  and then send it later.

Reply to Mail

- Select the message from the message list or open the
  message in its own window:

1. Click the Reply button [Reply].

   ✔ *The Reply submenu displays*

2. Click Reply to Sender to reply to the original sender only.

   OR

   Select Reply to Sender and All Recipients to send a reply to the
   sender and all other recipients of the original message.

- Selecting one of these options automatically inserts the recipient's name or e-mail address in the address fields.

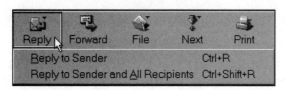

✔ *The Message Composition window opens, with the To, Cc, and Subject fields filled in for you.*

- Compose your reply as you would a new message.

To include a copy of the original message with your reply:

1. Select the original message from the message list.

2. Click the New Msg button New Msg on the Messenger toolbar.

3. Click the Quote button Quote on the Message Composition toolbar.

   ✔ *The entire message will be automatically inserted in the body of your new message. You can edit the original message and header text as you wish.*

4. When you are finished, click the Send button Send to send the message immediately.

Forward Mail

- To forward a message:

1. Select the message from the message list or open the message to forward.

2. Click the Forward button Forward from the toolbar.

   ✔ *The Message Composition window opens, with the Subject field filled in for you.*

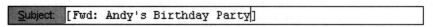

3. Type the e-mail address of the new recipient in the To field.

✔ *If the original message does not appear in*

the composition area, click the Quote button *on the Message Composition toolbar to insert it.*

4. Click in the composition area and edit the message as desired. You can also type any additional text you want to include with the forwarded message.

5. When you are done, click the Send button ![Send] to send the message immediately.

OR

Select File, Send Later to store the message in the Unsent Messages mailbox to be sent later.

OR

To save the reply as a draft to be edited and sent later, select Save Draft from the File menu.

Add Entries to the Personal Address Book

■ You can compile a personal Address Book to store e-mail addresses that you use often. Click on entries from the Address Book to insert an e-mail address automatically into the e-mail message header.

To add a name to the Address Book:

1. Click Communicator, Address Book.

✔ *The Address Book window displays.*

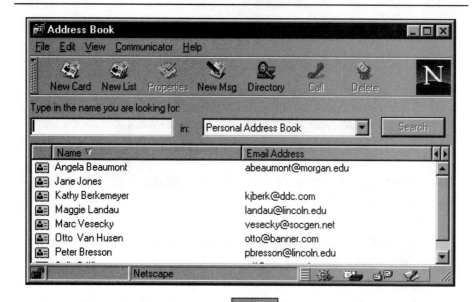

2. Click the New Card button 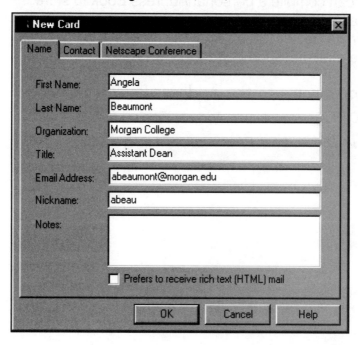 on the Address Book toolbar.

3. In the New Card box that appears, enter the recipient's first name, last name, organization, title, and e-mail address.

- In the Nickname field, if desired, type a unique nickname for the recipient. When addressing a message, you can use the recipient's nickname in the To field and Messenger will automatically fill in the full e-mail address.

- In the Notes field, type any notes you want to store about the recipient.

- Click the Contact tab, if desired, and enter the recipient's postal address and phone number.

4. Click [OK].

■ You can edit an address book entry at any time by double-clicking on the person's name in the Address Book window.

■ To add the name and address of the sender of a message you are reading:

- Click Message, Add to Address Book.

Add a name to the Address Book from the Add to Address Book submenu:

1. Right-click on unopened message.
2. Click Add to Address Book.
3. Click Sender to add the sender name to your address book.

   OR

   Click All to add all names from the addressee fields to the Address Book (e.g., everyone from the cc: field).

- The New Card dialog box opens, with the sender's name and e-mail address filled in for you. You can enter a nickname and any other information you want in the remaining fields.

Address a New Message Using the Personal Address Book

1. Click the New Msg button [New Msg] to open the Message Composition window.

2. Click on the Address button [Address] on the Message Composition toolbar and select a recipient(s) from the list in the Address Book window.

3. Double-click on the name from the list of addresses.

4. Click [OK] to close the Address Book. The name(s) are automatically inserted in the address field.

Netscape Messenger: 6

◆ Attached Files ◆ View File Attachments
◆ Save Attached Files ◆ Attach Files to Messages

Attached Files

- Sometimes an e-mail message will come with a separate file(s) attached. Messages containing attachments are indicated when you display a message and it contains a paperclip icon to the right of the message header. Attachments can be used when you want to send someone a document, a spreadsheet, a video clip, or any other type of file.

- With Messenger, you can view both plain text attachments and binary attachments. Binary files are files containing more than plain text (i.e., images, sound clips, and formatted text, such as spreadsheets and word processor documents).

- Almost any e-mail program can read plain text files. Binary files, however, must be decoded by the receiving e-mail program before they can be displayed in a readable form. When a binary attachment arrives, Messenger automatically recognizes and decodes it.

View File Attachments

- E-mail attachments are displayed in one of two ways.

View attachments Inline:

- If you select View, Attachments, Inline, you see the attachment in a separate attachment window below the message. If there is more than one attachment, you will see a series of sequential windows—one with the message and the other with the attachments.

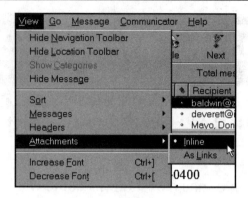

✔ *Only plain text, images, and Web page attachments can be viewed Inline.*

View attachments As Links:

- If you select View, Attachments, As Links, the window below the message displays an attachment box listing the details of the attachment. It also serves as a link to the attachment.

✔ *Viewing attachments as links reduces the time it takes to open a message on screen.*

- Click on the blue-highlighted text in the attachment box to display the attachment.

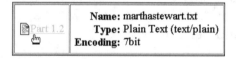

- You can right-click on the attachment icon portion of the attachment box to display a menu of mail options such as forwarding, replying, or deleting the message.

  - By right-clicking on the actual attachment, you can choose from several save options.

  - If you open a Web page attachment while online, you will connect to that Web site. If you are not online, the Web page will display fully formatted, but it will not be active.

- If an attached image displays as a link even after you select View, Attachments, Inline, it is probably because it is an image type that Messenger does not recognize. In this case, you need to install and/or open a plug-in or program with which to view the unrecognized image.

Save Attached Files

- You can save an attached file to your hard drive or disk for future use or reference.

To save an attachment:

1. Open the message containing the attachment to save.
2. If the attachment is in Inline view, convert it to a link (View, Attachments, As Links).
3. Right-click on the link and select Save Link As.

   OR

   Click on the link to open the attachment. Select File, Save As, or, if Messenger does not recognize the attachment's file type, click the Save File button in the Unknown File Type dialog box.

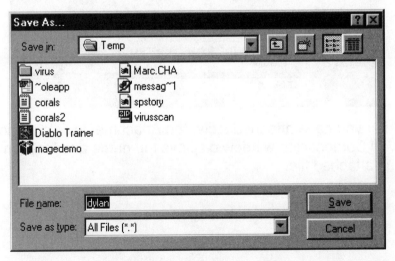

4. In the Save As dialog box that follows, click the Save in drop-down list box and select the drive and folder in which to save the file.
5. Click in the File name text box and type a name for the file.
6. Click Save.

Attach Files to Messages

- Any type of file can be sent as an attachment to an e-mail message—including text files, graphics, spreadsheets, and HTML documents.

To attach a file to an e-mail message:

1. Click the Attach button 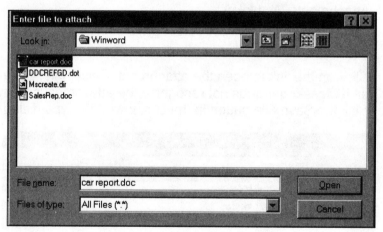 on the Message Composition toolbar, and select File from the drop-down menu that appears.
2. In the Enter file to attach dialog box that follows, click the Look in drop-down list box and select the drive and folder containing the file to attach.
3. Then select the file to attach and click Open.

- After you have attached a file, the Attachments field in the Mail Composition window displays the name and location of the attached file.

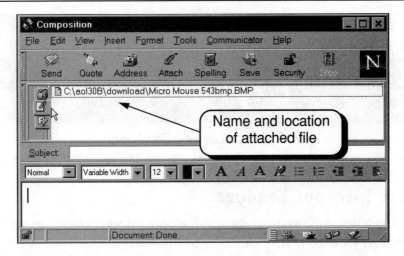

✔ *Messages containing attachments usually take longer to send than those without attachments. When attaching very large files or multiple files, you may want to zip (compress) the files before attaching them. To do so, both you and the recipient need a file compression program, such as WinZip or PKZip.*

■ Once you have attached the desired files and finished composing your message, you can send the e-mail, save it in the Unsent Messages folder for later delivery, or save it as a draft for later editing.

Microsoft Internet Explorer: 7

◆ Start Internet Explorer 4
◆ Internet Explorer Screen ◆ Exit Internet Explorer

Start Internet Explorer 4

- When you first install Internet Explorer and you are using the Active Desktop, you may see the message illustrated below when you turn on your computer. If you are familiar with Explorer 3, you may want to select 1 to learn the new features in Explorer 4. Select 2 to learn about Channels.

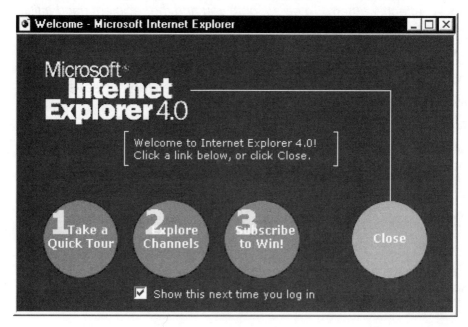

To start Internet Explorer:

- Click 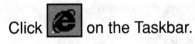 on the Desktop.

  OR

  Click [icon] on the Taskbar.

  OR

  Click the Start button [Start], then select Programs, Internet Explorer, and click Internet Explorer.

Internet Explorer Screen

- When you connect to the World Wide Web, the first screen that displays is called a home page. The home page is the first page of any World Wide Web site.

- You can change the first page that you see when you connect to Explorer.

To change the home page:

1. Click View, Internet Options.

2. Enter a new address in the Address text box.

   ✔ *The page that you see when you are connected may differ from the one illustrated below.*

3. Click [OK].

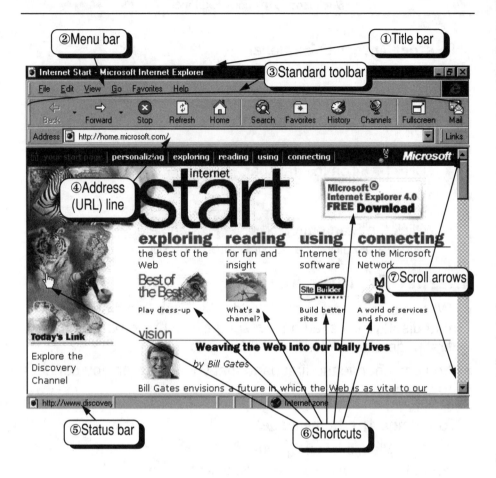

②Menu bar
①Title bar
③Standard toolbar
④Address (URL) line
⑦Scroll arrows
⑤Status bar
⑥Shortcuts

① **Title bar**   Displays the name of the program and the current Web page. You can minimize, restore, or close Explorer using the buttons on the right side of the Title bar.

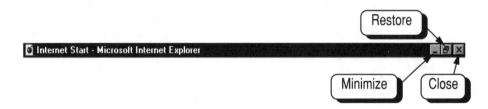

Restore

Minimize   Close

② **Menu bar**   Displays menus currently available, which provide drop-down lists of commands for executing Internet Explorer tasks.

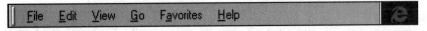

     The Internet Explorer button on the right side of the Menu bar rotates when action is occurring or information is being processed.

③ **Standard toolbar**   Displays frequently used commands.

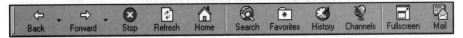

④ **Address (URL) line**   Displays the address of the current page. You can click here, type a new address, press Enter, and go to a new location (if it's an active Web site). You can also start a search from this line.

The Links bar contains links to various Microsoft sites. Drag the split bar to the left or somewhere else on the screen to display current Links. You can add or delete links.

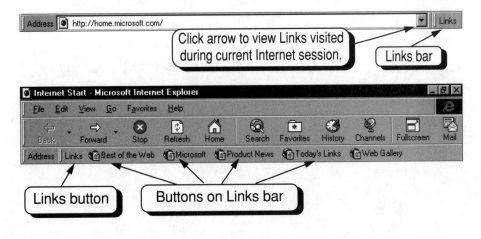

Click arrow to view Links visited during current Internet session.

Links bar

Links button   Buttons on Links bar

⑤ **Status bar**   Displays information about actions occurring on the page and the Security Level. Internet Security Properties lets you control content that is downloaded on to your computer.

⑥ **Shortcuts**   Click on shortcuts (also called hyperlinks) to move to other Web sites. Shortcuts are usually easy to recognize. They can be underlined text, text of different colors, "buttons" of various sizes and shapes, or graphics. You are pointing to a shortcut when the mouse pointer changes to a hand, and the full name of the Web site appears on the Status bar.

⑦ **Scroll arrows**   Scroll arrows are used to move the screen view, as in all Windows applications.

Exit Internet Explorer

- Exiting Internet Explorer and disconnecting from your service provider are two separate steps. It is important to remember that if you close Internet Explorer (or any other browser), you must also disconnect (or hang up) from your service provider. If you don't disconnect, you'll continue incurring any applicable charges.

Microsoft Internet Explorer: 8

◆ Standard Toolbar Buttons
◆ Open a Web Site from the Address Bar

Standard Toolbar Buttons

■ The Internet Explorer Standard toolbar displays frequently used commands. If the Standard toolbar is *not* visible when you start Explorer, open the View menu, select Toolbars, then select Standard Buttons.

Internet Explorer Toolbar and Functions

 Moves back through pages previously displayed. Back is available only if you have moved around among Web pages in the current Explorer session.

 Moves forward through pages previously displayed. Forward is available only if you have used the Back button.

 Interrupts the opening of a page that is taking too long to display.

 Reloads the current page.

 Returns you to your home page. You can change your home page to open to any Web site or a blank page (View, Internet Options, General).

 Allows you to select from a number of search services with a variety of options.

 Displays the Web sites that you have stored or bookmarked using the Favorites menu.

Displays links to Web sites that you have visited in previous days and weeks. You can change the number of days that sites are stored in your History folder (View, Internet Options, General).

Displays the list of current channels on the Explorer bar.

Conceals Menu, titles, Status bar, and Address bar to maximize your screen for viewing a Web page. Click it again to restore your screen.

Displays a drop-down menu with various Mail and News options. You will learn about Outlook Express e-mail options in Chapters 10-12.

Open a Web Site from the Address Bar

1. Click in the Address bar and start typing the address of the Web site you want to open.

2. If you have visited the site before, Internet Explorer will try to complete the address automatically. If it is the correct address, press Enter to go to it. If it is not the correct address, type over the suggested address that displayed on the line.

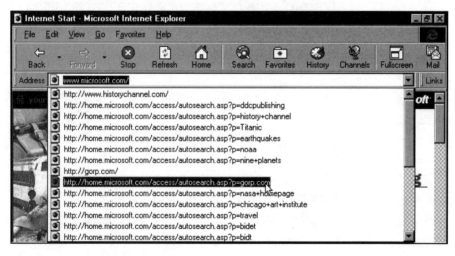

✔ *To turn off the AutoComplete feature, open the View menu,*
select Internet Options, and click the Advanced tab. Deselect
Use AutoComplete in the Browsing area of the dialog box.

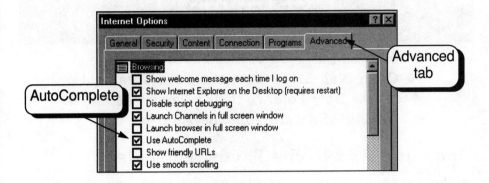

Microsoft Internet Explorer: 9

◆ Open and Add to the Favorites Folder
◆ Open Web Sites from the Favorites Folder
◆ Create New Folders in the Favorites Folder
◆ AutoSearch from the Address Bar

Open and Add to the Favorites Folder

■ As you spend more time exploring Web sites, you will find sites that you want to visit frequently. You can store shortcuts to these sites in the Favorites folder.

To add a site to the Favorites folder:

1. Go to the desired Web site.
2. Open the Favorites menu or right-click anywhere on the page and select Add To Favorites.

   ✔ *The Add Favorite dialog box appears*

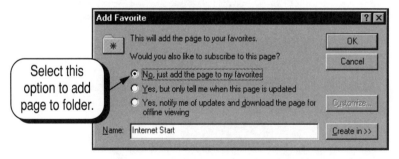

3. The name of the Page you have opened appears in the Name box. You may also choose to subscribe to a page. Subscribing to a page means you can schedule automatic updates to that site. Choose from the following options:

   ◆ No, just add the page to my favorites.

   ✔ *Choose this option to put a shortcut to the Web site in your Favorites folder.*

◆ <u>Y</u>es, but only tell me when this page is updated.

✔ *Explorer will alert you when an update to the site is available.*

◆ Yes, notify me of updates and <u>d</u>ownload the page for offline viewing

✔ *Explorer will automatically download and update to your computer.*

4. Click ▐ OK ▌ to add the Web address to the Favorites folder.

Open Web Sites from the Favorites Folder

■ Click the Favorites button 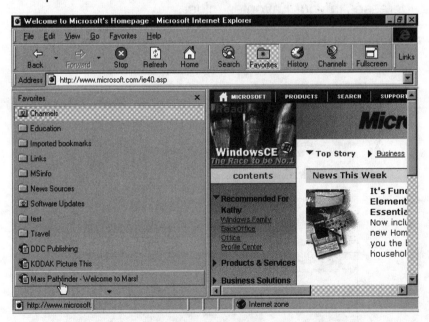 Favorites on the Standard toolbar to open Web sites from the Favorites folder. The Explorer bar will open on the left side of the Browser window.

■ Click on an address or open a folder and select a site. Close the Explorer bar by clicking the Close button ☒ or

the Favorites button ▐Favorites▌ on the toolbar.

- You can also open the Favorites menu and select a site from the list or from a folder.

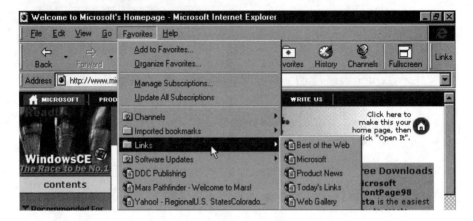

Create New Folders in the Favorites Folder

- You can create new folders before or after you have saved addresses in your Favorites folder.

To create a new folder:

1. Click Favorites and select Organize Favorites.
2. Click the Create New Folder button.
3. Type the name of the new folder and press Enter.

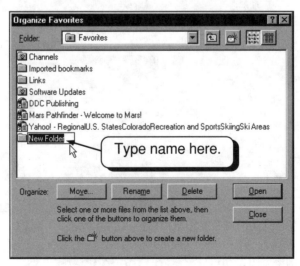

AutoSearch from the Address Bar

- In addition to displaying and entering addresses in the Address bar, you can use AutoSearch to perform a quick search directly from the Address bar.
- Click once in the Address bar and type *go, find,* or *?* and press the spacebar once. Enter the word or phrase you want to find and press Enter. For example, if you want to search for information about the year 2000, type *find the year 2000* on the Address bar and press Enter.

Address	find the year 2000

Outlook Express: 10

◆ Start Outlook Express
◆ Configure Outlook Express
◆ Outlook Express Main Window
◆ Retrieve New Messages ◆ The Mail Window
◆ Read Messages ◆ Delete a Message
◆ Print a Message ◆ Save a Message

Start Outlook Express

- Click the Mail icon on the Taskbar.

  OR

  Click <u>G</u>o, <u>M</u>ail.

✔ *Clicking the Mail icon from the Explorer main window may take you to the Microsoft Outlook organizational program. To use the more compact Outlook Express as your default mail program, click <u>V</u>iew, Internet <u>O</u>ptions from the Explorer main window. Click the Programs tab and choose Outlook Express from the <u>M</u>ail pull-down menu.*

✔ *If you downloaded Internet Explorer 4, be sure that you downloaded the standard version, which includes Outlook Express in addition to the Web browser.*

Configure Outlook Express

✔ *This section assumes that you have already set up an e-mail account with a service provider.*

- Establishing a modem connection and configuring your computer to send and receive mail can be frustrating. Don't be discouraged. What follows are steps that will get you connected, but some of the information may have to be supplied by your Internet Service Provider.

- Before you can use Outlook Express to send and receive e-mail, you must configure the program with your e-mail account information.

- You may have already filled in this information if you completed the Internet Connection Wizard when you started Internet Explorer for the first time. If not, you can enter the information by running the Internet Connection Wizard again.

Using Internet Connection Wizard

1. Launch Outlook Express.
2. Open the Tools menu, select Accounts.
3. Click the Mail tab.
4. Click Add and select Mail to start the Connection Wizard.

    ✔ *The Internet Connection Wizard will ask for information necessary to set up or add an e-mail account.*

5. Enter the name you want to appear on the "From" line in your outgoing messages. Click Next.

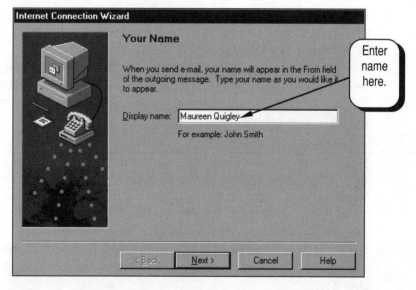

6. Type your e-mail address. This is the address that people use to send mail to you. Click Next.
7. Enter the names of your incoming and outgoing mail servers. Check with your Internet Service Provider if you do not know what they are. Click Next.

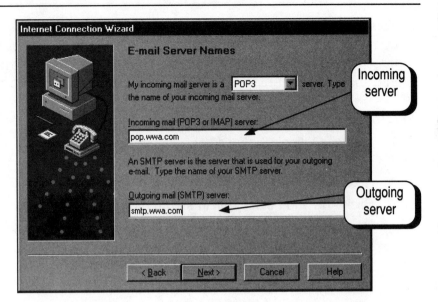

8. Enter the logon name and password that your ISP requires for you to access your mail. Again, if you are not sure about this information, contact your ISP. Click Next.

9. Enter a name for your e-mail account. The name you enter will appear when you open the Accounts list on the Tools menu in Outlook Express. It can be any name that you choose. Click Next.

10. Select the type of connection you are using to reach the Internet. If you are connecting through a phone line, you will need to have a dial-up connection. If you have an existing connection, click Next and select from the list of current connections.

11. Select Use an existing dial-up connection, or select Create a new dial-up connection and follow the directions to create a new one.

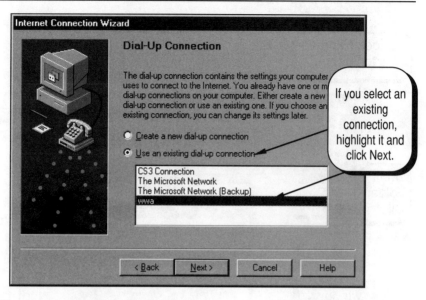

12. If you select Use an existing dial-up connection, click Finish in the last window to save the settings.

✔ *You should then be able to launch Outlook Express and send and receive mail and attachments.*

Outlook Express Main Window

- After you launch Outlook Express, the main Outlook Express window opens by default. You can access any e-mail function from this window.

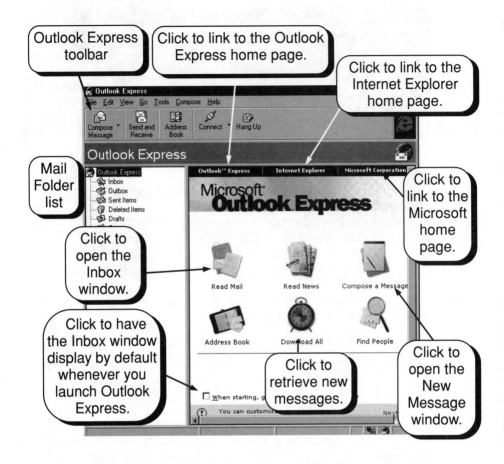

The following callouts appear in the figure:

- Outlook Express toolbar
- Click to link to the Outlook Express home page.
- Click to link to the Internet Explorer home page.
- Click to link to the Microsoft home page.
- Mail Folder list
- Click to open the Inbox window.
- Click to have the Inbox window display by default whenever you launch Outlook Express.
- Click to retrieve new messages.
- Click to open the New Message window.

■ Descriptions of items in the main window follow below:

- The Mail Folder list displays in the left column of the window, with the Outlook Express main folder selected. To view the contents of a different folder, click on the desired folder in the folder list.

- Shortcuts to different e-mail functions are located in the center of the window. Click on a shortcut to access the indicated task or feature.

- Hyperlinks to Microsoft home pages are located at the top of the window. Click on a link to connect to the indicated home page.

- The Outlook Express toolbar displays buttons for commonly used commands. Note that each button contains an image and text that describes the button function. Clicking any of these buttons will activate the indicated task immediately.

Retrieve New Messages

- You can retrieve new mail from any Outlook Express window.

1. Click the Send and Receive button on the toolbar.

2. In the Connection dialog box that displays, enter your ISP user name in the <u>U</u>ser Name text box and your password in the <u>P</u>assword text box. Click OK. (If you do not know your user name or password, contact your ISP.)

✔ *You must re-enter your password each time you reconnect to the Internet unless you set Outlook Express to save your password permanently. To do so, select the Save <u>P</u>assword check box in the connection dialog box and click OK.*

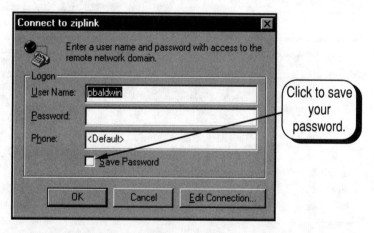

3. Once you are connected to the Internet and Outlook Express is connected to your ISP mail server, new mail messages will begin downloading from your ISP mail server.

✔ *A dialog box displays the status of your retrieval.*

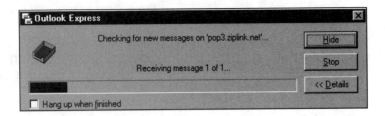

The Mail Window

- After retrieving new messages, Outlook Express stores them in the Inbox folder.

- To view your new messages, you must open the Mail window and display the contents of the Inbox folder.

1. Click the Read Mail shortcut [Read Mail] in the Outlook Express main window.

2. The Mail window opens with the Inbox folder displayed. A description of the items in the Mail window appears on the following page.

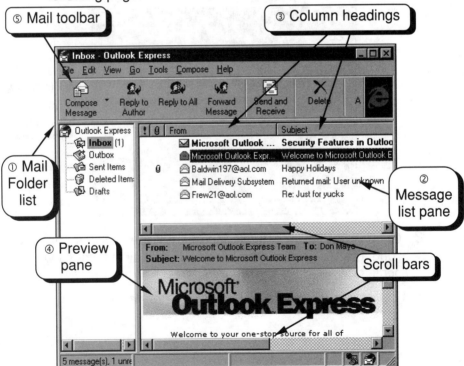

✔ *In the message list, unread messages are displayed in bold text with a sealed envelope icon* *. Messages that have been read are listed in regular text with an open envelope icon* *.*

① The Mail Folder list displays the currently selected message folder, the contents of which are displayed in the mail list. Click on another folder to display its contents in the mail list.

② The message list pane displays a header for each of the messages contained in the currently selected mail folder.

③ Column headings list the categories of information included in each message header, such as subject, from, and date received.

④ The preview pane displays the content of the message currently selected from the message list. You can show/hide the preview pane by selecting View, Layout and clicking on the Use preview pane check box.

⑤ The Mail toolbar displays command buttons for working with messages. These commands vary depending on the message folder currently displayed (Inbox, Sent, Outbox, etc.).

Read Messages

✔ *You do not have to be online to read e-mail. You can reduce your online time if you disconnect from your ISP after retrieving your messages and read them offline.*

■ You must have the Mail window open and the mail folder containing the message to read displayed.

To read messages:

• To read a message in the preview pane, click on the desired message header in the message list. If the message does not appear, select View, Layout, Use preview pane.

OR

To open and read a message in a separate window, double-click on the desired message header in the message list.

✔ *The Message window opens displaying the Message toolbar and the contents of the selected message.*

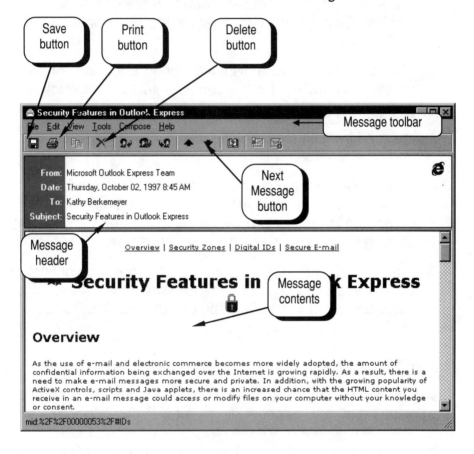

To close the Message window:

* Click File, Close.

OR

Click on the Close button (X) in the upper-right corner of the window.

✔ *Use the scroll bars in the Message window or the preview pane to view hidden parts of a displayed message. Or, press the down arrow key to scroll down through the message.*

To read the next unread message:

- Select View, Next, Next Unread Message.

  OR

  If you are viewing a message in the Message window, click the Next button [▼] on the Message toolbar.

■ Once you have read a message, it remains stored in the Inbox folder until you delete it or file it in another folder.

Delete a Message

1. Select the desired header from the message list in the Mail window.

2. Click the Delete button [✕ Delete] in the Mail toolbar, or select Edit, Delete.

   OR

1. Open the desired message in the Message window.

2. Click the Delete button [✕] on the Message toolbar.

✔ *To select more than one message from the message list to delete, press the Ctrl button while you click each message header.*

Print a Message

1. Select the message you want to print from the message list in the Mail window or open the message in the Message window.

2. Select Print from the File menu.

3. In the Print dialog box that opens, select the desired print options and click OK.

■ You can send the message to the printer using the most recently used print settings by opening the message in the Message window and clicking the Print button [🖨] on the Message toolbar.

Save a Message

1. Open the desired message in the Message window and click the Save button 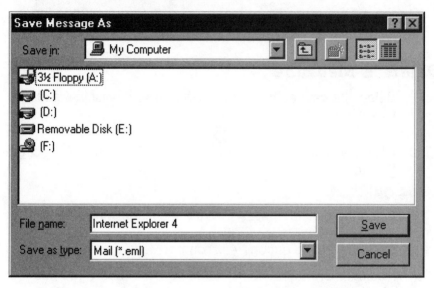 on the Message toolbar.

2. In the Save Message As dialog box that opens, click the Save in drop-down list box and select the drive and folder in which to store the message file.

3. Click in the File name box and enter a name for the message.
4. Click Save.

Outlook Express: 11

◆ Compose New Messages ◆ Send Messages
◆ Reply to Mail ◆ Forward Mail
◆ Add Entries to the Personal Address Book
◆ Address a New Message Using the Personal
Address Book

Compose New Messages

■ You can compose an e-mail message in Outlook Express online or offline. When composing an e-mail message online, you can send the message immediately after creating it.

■ When composing a message offline, you will need to store the message in your Outbox folder until you are online and can send it. (See **Send Messages** on page 60.)

To create a message:

1. Open the New Message window.

2. Click the Compose Message button on the toolbar in either the Mail window or the Main window.

   ✔ *The New Message window displays.*

3. In the New Message window, type the e-mail address(es) of the message recipient(s) in the To field.

   ✔ *If you type the first few characters of a name or e-mail address that is saved in your Address Book, Outlook Express will automatically complete it for you.*

   OR

   Click the Index Card icon in the To field or the Address Book button on the New Message toolbar and select an address to insert from your personal Address Book. (See page 64 for information on using the Address Book.)

   ✔ *If you are sending the message to multiple recipients, insert a comma or semicolon between each recipient's address.*

4. After inserting the address(es) in the To field, you may click in either of the following fields and enter the recipient information indicated:

CC (Carbon Copy)	The e-mail addresses of people who will receive copies of the message.
BCC (Blind Carbon Copy)	Same as CC, except these names will not appear anywhere in the message, so other recipients will not know that the person(s) listed in the BCC field received a copy.

5. Click in the Subject field and type the subject of the message. An entry in this field is required.

6. Type your message in the blank composition area below the Subject field.

    ✔ *You can check the spelling of your message by selecting Spelling from the Tools menu and responding to the prompts that follow.*

Send Messages

- Once you have created a message, you have three choices:
  - to send the message immediately
  - to store the message in the Outbox folder to be sent later
  - to save the message in the Drafts folder to be edited and sent later

To send a message immediately:

✔ *In order to send messages immediately, you must first select Options from the Tools menu in the Mail window. Then click on the Send tab and select the Send messages immediately check box. If this option is not selected, clicking the Send button will not send a message immediately, but will send the message to your Outbox until you perform the Send and Receive task.*

1. Click the Send button [✉ Send] on the New Message toolbar.

    OR

    Click File, Send Message.

2. Outlook Express then connects to your ISP's mail server and sends out the new message. If the connection to the mail server is successful, the sending mail icon displays in the lower-right corner of the status bar until the transmittal is complete.

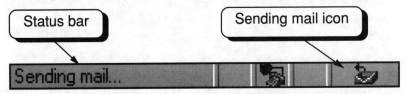

Status bar

Sending mail icon

Sending mail...

- Sometimes, however, Outlook Express cannot immediately connect to the mail server and instead has to store the new message in the Outbox for later delivery. When this happens, the sending mail icon does not appear, and the number next to your Outbox folder increases by one **Outbox [1]**.

- Outlook Express does not automatically reattempt to send a message after a failed connection. Instead, you need to send the message manually from the Outbox (see **To send messages from your Outbox folder** below).

To store a message in your Outbox folder for later delivery:

1. Select File, Send Later in the New Message window.

    ✔ *The Send Mail prompt displays, telling you that the message will be stored in our Outbox folder.*

2. Click OK.

    ✔ *The message is saved in the Outbox.*

To send messages from your Outbox folder:

- Click on the Send and Receive button Send and Receive on the toolbar.

    OR

    Click Tools, Send and Receive, All Accounts.

✔ When you use the Send and Receive command, Outlook Express sends out all messages stored in the Outbox and automatically downloads any new mail messages from the mail server.

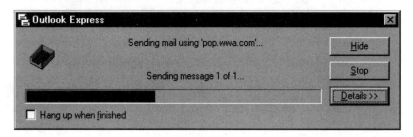

Reply to Mail

- In Outlook Express, you can reply to a message automatically, without having to enter the recipient's name or e-mail address.

- When replying, you have a choice of replying to the author and all recipients of the original message or to the author only.

To reply to the author and all recipients:

1. Select the message you want to reply to from the message list in the Mail window.

2. Click the Reply to All button [Reply to All] on the Mail toolbar.

To reply to the author only:

- Click the Reply to Author button [Reply to Author] on the Mail toolbar.

- Once you have selected a reply command, the New Message window opens with the address fields and the Subject filled in for you.

  ✔ You can access all of the mail send commands by right-clicking on the message in the Message list.

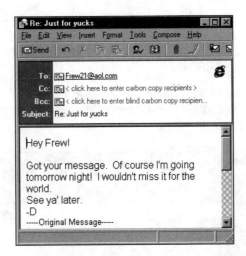

- The original message is automatically included in the body of your response. To turn off this default insertion, select Options from the Tools menu, click on the Send tab, deselect the Include message in reply check box, and click OK.

- To compose your reply, click in the composition area and type your text as you would in a new message.

- When you are done, click the Send button ⌷Send on the New Message toolbar to send the message immediately. Or, select Send Later from the File menu to store the message in the Outbox folder for later delivery. To save the reply as a draft to be edited and sent later, select Save from the File menu.

Forward Mail

- There are times when you will want to forward mail that you have received.

   1. Select the message to forward from the message list in the Mail window.

   2. Click the Forward Message button on the Mail toolbar.

      ✔ *The New Message window opens with the original message displayed and the Subject field filled in for you.*

3. Fill in the e-mail address information by either typing each address or selecting the recipients from your Address Book. (See **Address a New Message Using the Personal Address Book** on page 66.)

✔ *If you are forwarding the message to multiple recipients, insert a comma or semicolon between each recipient's address.*

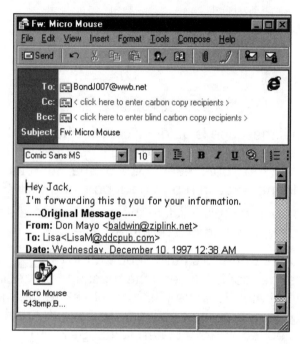

4. Click in the composition area and type any text you wish to send with the forwarded message.

5. When you are done, click the Send button ▣Send on the New Message toolbar to send the message immediately.

OR

Select Send Later from the File menu to store the message in the Outbox folder for later delivery.

Add Entries to the Personal Address Book

■ In Outlook Express, you can use the Windows Address Book to store e-mail addresses. You can then use the Address Book to find and automatically insert addresses when creating new messages.

To add an entry to the Address Book:

1. Click the Address Book button ![Address Book] on the toolbar in the Mail window or the Main window.

    ✔ *The Address Book window opens.*

2. Click the New Contact button ![New Contact] on the Address Book toolbar.

    ✔ *The Contact Properties dialog box displays.*

3. In the Properties dialog box, type the First, Middle, and Last names of the new contact in the appropriate text boxes.

4. Type the contact's e-mail address in the Add new text box and then click the Add button.

    ✔ *You can repeat this procedure if you wish to list additional e-mail addresses for the contact.*

5. In the Nickname text box, you can enter a unique nickname for the contact.

    ✔ *When addressing a new message, you can type the nickname in the To field, rather than typing the entire address, and Outlook Express will automatically complete the address.*

To add an Address Book entry from an e-mail message:

-   You can automatically add the name and address of the sender of a message.

    1. Open the message in the Message window.

    2. Right-click on the sender's name in the To field.

    3. Select Add to Address Book from the shortcut menu.

-   You can also set Outlook Express to add the address of recipients automatically when you reply to a message.

    ♦ Select Options from the Tools menu and select the Automatically put people I reply to in my Address Book check box on the General tab.

✔ *You can edit an Address Book entry at any time by double-clicking on the person's name in the contact list in the Address Book window.*

Address a New Message Using the Personal Address Book

1. Click the Select Recipients button 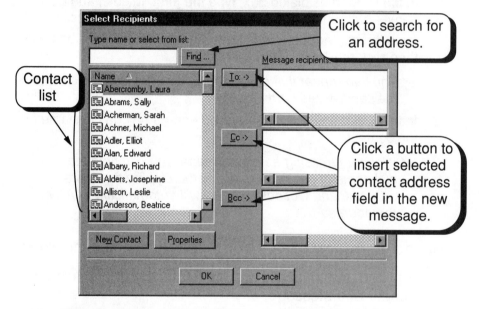 on the New Message toolbar.

2. In the Select Recipients dialog box that follows, select the address to insert from the contact list.

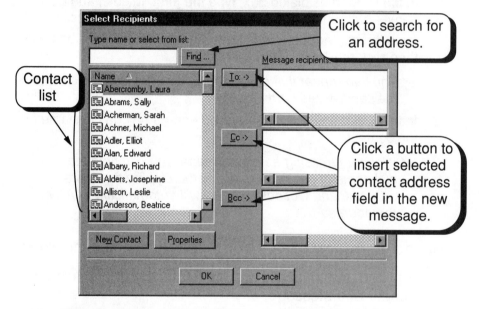

3. Click the button for the field in which you want to insert the address (To, Cc, or Bcc).

4. Click OK to return to the New Message window when you are finished.

Outlook Express: 12

◆ View Attached Files ◆ Save Attached Files
◆ Attach Files to a Message

View Attached Files

■ Sometimes e-mail messages come with separate files attached. Messages containing attachments show a paperclip icon to the left of the message header.

■ If the selected message is displayed in the preview pane, a larger paper clip attachment icon will appear to the right of the header at the top of the preview pane.

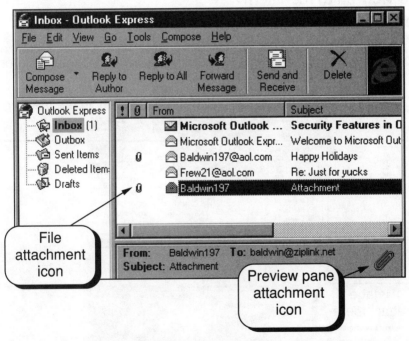

■ If you open the selected message in its own window, an attachment icon will appear in a separate pane below the message.

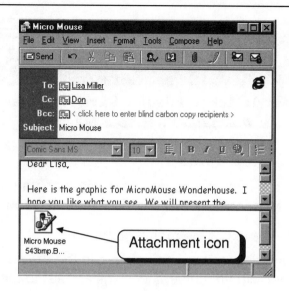

To view an attachment:

1. Open the folder containing the desired message in the Mail window.
2. Select the message containing the desired attachment(s) from the message list to display it in the preview pane.

   ✔ *If the attachment is an image, it will display in the message.*

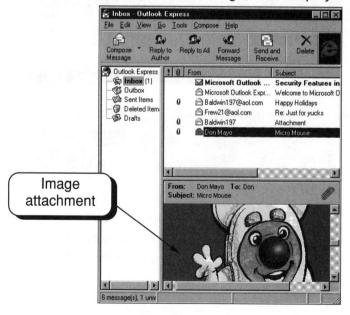

✔ *If the image does not display, click Tools, Options, click the Read tab, select the Automatically show picture attachments in messages check box, and click OK.*

■ Other types of attachments, such as programs, word processor documents, or media clips, do not display in the message, but have to be opened in a separate window.

To open an attachment in a separate window:

1. Click on the attachment icon 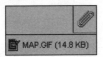 in the preview pane. A button will display with the file name and size of the attachment.

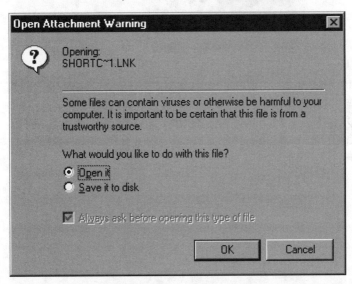

2. Click on this button.
3. If the Open Attachment Warning dialog box displays, select the desired option and click OK.

✔ *If you are not sure of the source of the attachment, you may want to save the attachment to a disk and run it through an anti-virus program.*

- Outlook Express will open the attached file or play the attached media clip.

- If the attached file does not open, Outlook Express does not recognize the file type of the attached file. Your computer may not contain the necessary plug-in or application to view it.

- To view an unrecognized attachment, you have to install and/or open the application or plug-in needed to view it.

Save Attached Files

- If desired, you can save an attached file to your hard drive or disk for future use or reference.

To save an attachment:

1. Select Save Attachments from the File menu, and select the attachment to save from the submenu that displays.

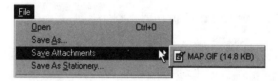

   OR

   Right-click on the attachment icon in the Message window and select the Save As option.

2. In the Save As dialog box that follows, click the Save in drop-down list box and select the drive and folder in which to save the file.

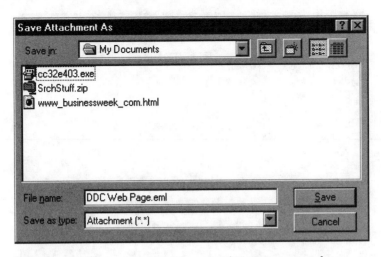

3. Click in the File name text box and type a name for the file.

4. Click Save.

Attach Files to a Message

■ You can attach a file to an e-mail message.

   ✔ *When attaching very large files or multiple files, you may want to zip (compress) the files before attaching them. To do so, both you and the recipient need a file compression program, such as WinZip or PKZip.*

To add an attachment:

1. Click the Insert File button 📎 on the New Message toolbar.

   OR

   Click Insert, File Attachment.

2. In the Insert Attachment dialog box that appears, click the Look in drop-down list box and select the drive and folder containing the file to attach. Then select the file and click Attach.

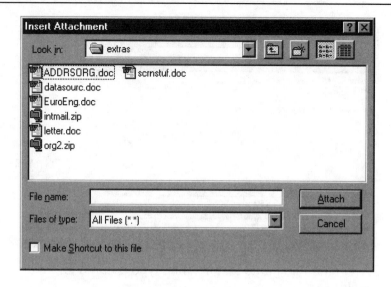

✔ The attachment will appear as an icon in the body of the message.

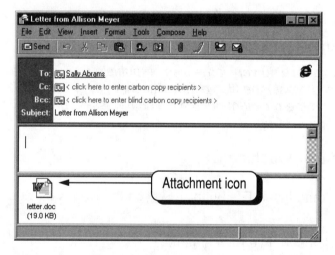

Attachment icon

✔ You can add multiple attachments by repeating the procedure as many times as you like.

✔ Before you send a message containing an attachment, you should make sure the recipient's e-mail program can read the attachment.

America Online: 13

About America Online

- America Online (AOL) is an all-purpose online service. Unlike Netscape Navigator or Microsoft Internet Explorer, AOL is not an Internet browser, yet you can browse the Internet using AOL navigation features.

- Unlike Internet browsers, AOL does not require a separate Internet Service Provider for Internet access, nor does it require a separate mail server connection to access e-mail from the AOL Mail Center.

Start America Online 4.0

1. Click the AOL icon ▲ on your desktop. This icon should display on your desktop after you install AOL.

   OR

   Click the Start button 🔲 Start , Programs, America Online, America Online 4.0.

2. Make sure your screen name is displayed in the Select Screen Name box and type your password in the Enter Password box.

3. Click the Sign On button SIGN ON to connect to the AOL server.

The AOL Home Page, Menu, and Toolbar

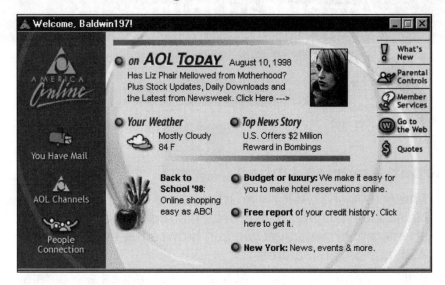

- After you log on to America Online, you will see a series of screens. The final first screen you see is the AOL home page or start page. The AOL home page contains links to daily AOL featured areas and constant AOL areas such as *Channels* and *What's New*. You can also access your mailbox from the home page.

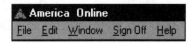

- The AOL menu displays currently available options. Click the menu item to display a drop-down list of links to AOL areas and basic filing, editing, and display options.

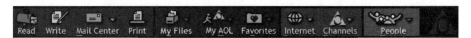

- The AOL toolbar contains buttons for AOL's most commonly used commands. Choosing a button activates the indicated task immediately.

	You have new mail if the flag on the mailbox is in the up position. Click to display your mailbox.
	Click to compose new mail messages.
	Click to read new, old, or sent mail; to set mail preferences; and to activate Flashsessions.
	Click to open the Print dialog box, where you can select from the standard print options.
	Click to access the Personal Filing Cabinet, where you can store e-mail messages, Newsgroup messages, and other files.
	Click to set AOL preferences, check personalized stock portfolios, read news and current events, set parental controls, passwords, and Buddy lists.
	Click this button to create links or shortcuts to your favorite Web sites or AOL areas.
	Click to connect to the Web, Internet directories, and Newsgroups.
	Click to access AOL's 21 channels, AOL areas, and Web site connections.
	Click to access the AOL Community Center, Chat Rooms, and meet the stars in the Live chat forum.
	Click to move to keywords or information entered on the URL line.
	Each AOL area has a keyword. Enter the keyword for immediate access to the desired AOL area.

AOL Help

- AOL offers extensive Help so that you can learn to use AOL effectively.
- To access Help, click Help and the help topic of choice from the menu.

Exit AOL

- To exit AOL, click the Close button ⊠ in the upper-right corner of the AOL screen.

  OR

  Click Sign Off, Sign Off on the menu bar.

  OR

  Click File, Exit.

America Online: 14

◆ Access the Internet from AOL
◆ Open a Wold Wide Web Site
◆ The AOL Browser Screen ◆ Stop a Load or Search

Access the Internet from AOL

- Click the Internet button **Internet** on the AOL main screen.

  OR

  Press Ctrl+K, type the word *internet* in the Keyword box and press Enter.

  ✔ *The Internet Connection window displays.*

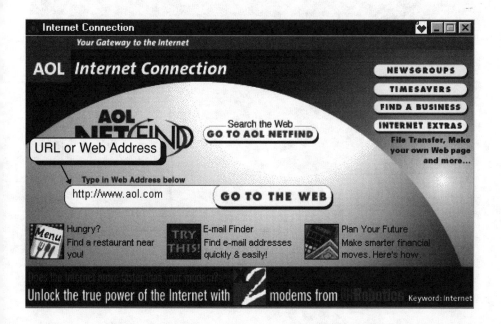

Open a World Wide Web Site

- If you know the Web address (URL), type it into the Type in Web Address below box and click the GO TO THE WEB button **GO TO THE WEB** or press Enter. If the Web address is correct, you will be connected to the Web site.

- If you wish to search the Internet, click the GO TO AOL NETFIND button **GO TO AOL NETFIND**.

The AOL Browser Screen

- Once you are connected to the Web, the screen below displays.

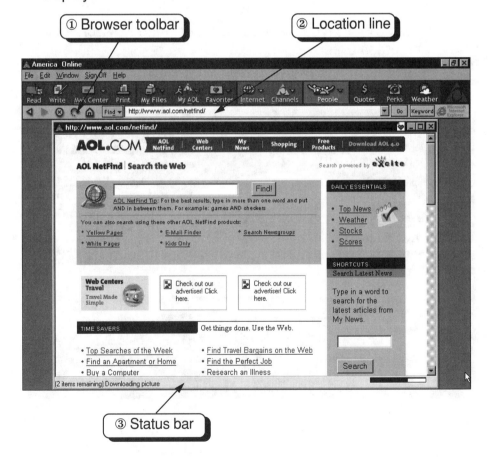

① Browser toolbar

② Location line

③ Status bar

① Browser toolbar

- The AOL Browser toolbar will help you navigate through sites you visit on the Web. Buttons on the Browser toolbar also connect you to search and Internet preference areas.

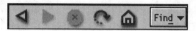

◁	Moves back through pages previously displayed.
▷	Moves forwards through pages previously displayed.
↻	Reloads an image that has been downloaded or restarts a load that has been interrupted. Since the image is stored in the computer's memory, it reloads much faster.
⊗	Stops the loading of a Web page.
⌂	Returns to your home page.
Find ▼	Go here to search the AOL directory using keywords or phrases, to search the Internet, or to find AOL access numbers.

② Location line

- AOL stores each Web address you visit during each AOL session. If you wish to return to an address you have visited during the current session, you can click the location box arrow and click the address from the drop-down list.

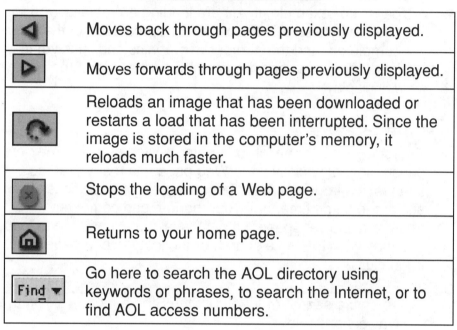

③ Status bar

Transferring document (443200 of 1000000 bytes)...

Status Message

- The Status bar, located at the bottom of the screen, is a helpful indicator of the progress of the loading of a Web page. For example, if you are loading a Web site, you will see the byte size of the page, the percentage of the task completed, and the number of graphics and links yet to load. In many cases the time it will take to load the page will display.

Stop a Load or Search

- Searching for information or loading a Web page can be time consuming, especially if the Web page has many graphic images, if a large number of people are trying to access the site at the same time, or if your modem and computer operate at slower speeds. If data is taking a long time to load, you may wish to stop a search or the loading of a page or large file.

  - To stop a search or load click the Stop button [×] on the Navigation toolbar.

  - If you decide to continue the load after clicking the Stop button [×], click the Reload button [↻].

America Online: 15

Favorite Places

- A Favorite Place listing is a bookmark that you create containing the title, URL, and direct link to a Web page or AOL area that you may want to revisit.

- The AOL Favorite Place feature allows you to maintain a record of Web sites in your Favorite Places file so that you can return to them easily.

Add Favorite Places

- There are several ways to mark an AOL area or Web site and save it as a Favorite Place. Once the page is displayed:

   1. Click the Favorite Place icon 💟 on the Web site or AOL area title bar.

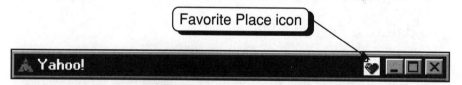

Favorite Place icon

   2. Click on one of three options that display:

   Add to Favorites

   ✔ *The site will automatically be added to your Favorite Places list.*

   OR

   Insert in Instant Message

   ✔ *The site will automatically generate an Instant Message screen with a link to the site inserted.*

OR

Insert in Mail

✔ *The site will automatically generate an e-mail composition screen with a link to the site inserted. Complete this as you would any e-mail message.*

OR

Display the Web page to add, right-click anywhere on the page and select Add to Favorites from the shortcut menu.

View Favorite Places

- You can view the Favorite Places file by clicking the Favorites button Favorites on the AOL toolbar and selecting Favorite Places. Click on any listing from the list to go directly to that page.

- The details of any Favorite Place listing can be viewed or modified by using the buttons on the Favorite Places screen.

Delete Favorite Places

- You may wish to delete a Favorite Place if a Web site no longer exists or an AOL area no longer interests you.

To delete a Favorite Place:

1. Click the Favorite Places button Favorites on the toolbar.
2. Click Favorite Places.
3. Click on the listing to delete.

4. Click the Delete button Delete from the Favorite Places screen.

   OR

   Right-click on the listing and select Delete from the pop-up menu.

   OR

   Press the Delete key.

5. Click [Yes] to confirm the deletion.

AOL History List

- While you move back and forth within a Web site, AOL automatically records each page location. The History is only temporary and is deleted when you sign off. AOL areas are not recorded in the History list.

- To view the History list, click on the arrow at the end of the URL line. You can use History to jump back or forward to recently viewed pages by clicking on the page from the list.

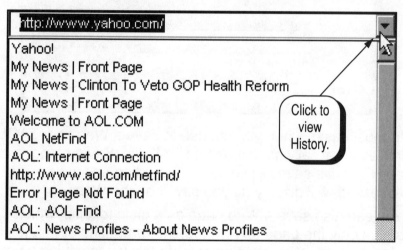

Save Web Pages

- When you find a Web page with information that you would like to keep for future reference or to review later offline, you can save it.

To save a Web page:

1. Click File, Save.
2. Type a filename in the File name box.

   ✔ When you save a Web page, often the current page name appears in the File name box. You can use this name or type a new one.

3. Choose the drive and folder in which to store the file from the Save in drop-down list.

4. Click Save.

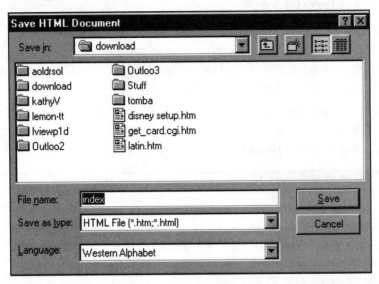

- In most cases when you choose to save a Web page, AOL will automatically save it as an HTML file. Saving a page as an HTML file saves the original formatting and, when accessed, will display as you saw it on the Web.

- You can also save a Web page as a plain text file, which saves only the page text without the formatting or images and placeholders. You might want to do this when saving a very large file, such as a literary work or multiple-page article. To save in plain text format, click the Save as type down arrow in the Save As dialog box and select plain text from the list.

- You can view a saved Web page by clicking File, Open. In the Open a file dialog box, choose the location from the Look in drop-down list and double-click the file name.

Print Web Pages

■ One of the many uses of the Internet is to find and print information.

To print a Web page, display it and do the following:

1. Click the Print button ▣ Print on the AOL toolbar.

   OR

   Click <u>P</u>rint on the <u>F</u>ile menu.
2. In the Print dialog box that displays, select the desired print options and click OK.

■ In most cases, the Web page will be printed in the format shown in the Web page display.

America Online E-mail: 16

◆ Read New Mail ◆ Compose a New Mail Message
◆ Send Messages ◆ Reply to Mail
◆ Forward Mail ◆ AOL Mail Help

Read New Mail

■ There are several ways to know whether you have new mail in your mailbox. If your computer has a sound card and speakers, you will hear "You've Got Mail" when you successfully connect to AOL. The link is replaced by the You Have Mail link, and the mailbox button on the main screen has the flag in the up position .

To display and read new and unread mail:

1. Click the You Have Mail button on the AOL main screen.

   OR

   Click the Read button on the main screen toolbar.

   OR

   Press Ctrl+R.

   ✔ *The New Mail list displays new and unread mail for the screen name used for this session. If you have more than one screen name, you must sign on under each name to retrieve new mail. Click S̲ign Off, Switch Scree̲n Names to switch names without logging off AOL.*

   ✔ *New and Unread e-mail messages remain on the AOL mail server for approximately 27 days before being deleted by AOL. If you want to save a message to your hard disk, click F̲ile, S̲ave As and choose a location for the message. By default the message will be saved to the Download folder.*

✔ *You can set up AOL to save read messages up to seven days by clicking the My AOL button from the toolbar. Click Preferences, and then click the Mail button 🔖. Set the number of desired days in the Keep My Old Mail Online option box.*

2. To read a message, double-click on it from the New Mail list.

Compose a New Mail Message

1. Click Mail Center, Write Mail.

   OR

   Click the Write button Write on the main screen toolbar.

   OR

   Press Ctrl+M.

   ✔ *The Compose Mail screen displays.*

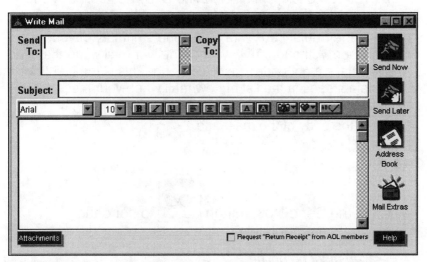

2. Fill in the e-mail address(es) in the Send To box of the Compose Mail screen.

   OR

   Click the Address Book button ![Address Book] on the right side of the Write Mail screen and double-click on an entry from your Address Book to insert an address automatically in the address field. (See page 91 for more information on your Address Book.)

+ If you are sending the same message to multiple recipients, fill in the Copy To (Carbon Copy) box with the e-mail addresses of recipients who will receive a copy of this message. These names will display to all recipients of the message.

✔ *Multiple addresses must be separated with a comma.*

+ If you want to send a Blind Copy—copies of a message sent to others but whose names are not visible to the main or other recipients, enclose the address in parenthesis, for example: (joes@ddcpub.com) or click the Blind Copy button when inserting addresses from the Address Book.

✔ *You can enclose multiple Blind Copy addresses in one set of parentheses, e.g., (joes@ddcpub.com, Zacz).*

3. Fill in the Subject box with a one-line summary of your message. Although AOL will now deliver mail without a heading it's always a good idea to include one. This is the first thing the recipient sees in the list of new mail when your message is delivered.

4. Fill in the body of the message.

Send Messages

* Click the Send Now button ![Send Now] to send the message immediately.

   ✔ *You must be online.*

   OR

   Click the Send Later button ![Send Later] to send a message later that you have composed offline.

88

Reply to Mail

- You can reply to mail messages while online or compose replies to e-mail offline to send later.

To reply to e-mail:

1. Click the Reply button from the displayed message screen. If the message has been sent to more than one person, you can send your response to each recipient of the message by clicking the Reply to All button. The addresses of the sender and, if desired, all recipients will be automatically inserted into the address fields.

   ✔ *To include part or all of the original message in your Reply, select the contents of the original message to be included in quotation marks in your message. Then click the Reply button to begin your reply.*

   ✔ *You can select mail preferences like the quotation style by clicking My AOL, Preferences, and the Mail icon.*

2. Click the Send Now button if you are online and want to send the reply immediately or click the Send Later button.

Forward Mail

- There are times when you may want to send mail you receive to someone else.

To forward e-mail:

1. Click the Forward button [Forward] from the displayed message screen and fill in the address(es) of the recipients of the forwarded message. The Subject heading from the original message is automatically inserted into the subject heading box.

2. Click the Send Now button [Send Now] if you are online and want to send the reply immediately or click the Send Later button [Send Later].

AOL Mail Help

- For answers to many of your basic e-mail questions, click Mail Center, Mail Center, and click on the Help button [HELP] on the Mail Center screen.

America Online E-mail: 17

◆ Add Entries to the Address Book
◆ Enter an Address Using the Address Book
◆ Delete an Address Book Entry

Add Entries to the Address Book

- Once you start sending e-mail, you may be surprised at how many people you begin to communicate with online. An easy way to keep track of e-mail addresses is to enter them into the Address Book. Once an e-mail address entry has been created, you can automatically insert it into the address fields.

To create Address Book entries:

1. Click Mail Center, Address Book.

   ✔ *The Address Book dialog box displays.*

2. Click the New Person button ![New Person] from the Address Book screen.

   ✔ *The New Person dialog box displays.*

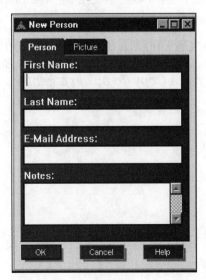

3. Enter the first and last name or a nickname (e.g., JohnV). The name(s) you enter in these boxes is how the entry will appear in the Address Book list.

4. Press the Tab key to move to the E-Mail Address box and enter the complete e-mail address of the recipient.

   ✔ *When entering the address of an AOL member, you do not need to enter the @aol.com domain information. Enter only their screen name as the e-mail address. For all other Address Book entries you must enter the entire address.*

5. Include any information you might want to remember about the person in the Notes box.

6. Click [OK].

Enter an Address Using the Address Book

1. Place the cursor in the address field.

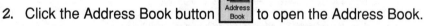

2. Click the Address Book button [Address Book] to open the Address Book.

3. Double-click the name or names from the Address Book list to insert in the Send To or Copy To address box using the appropriate buttons from the Address Book screen.

   ✔ *Unlike addresses entered in the Send To or Copy To address fields, addresses entered using the Blind Copy feature will not be visible to other recipients of the e-mail*

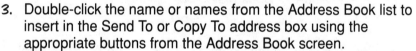

   message. Clicking the Blind Copy button [Blind Copy] after selecting an address from the Address Book inserts the address in the Copy To box in parentheses.

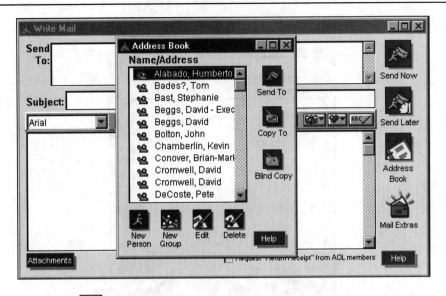

4. Click ✗ in the upper right-hand corner to close the Address Book.

To add an Address Book entry
from mail received:

1. Open the e-mail message.

2. Click the Add Address button Add Address from the message screen.

3. Enter the first and last name of the sender. The information entered into these fields will appear in the Address Book listing.

4. Notice that the e-mail address has been filled in for you.

5. Enter any information you may want to remember about the person in the Notes box.

6. Click OK .

To create a Group Entry:

1. To enter a Group listing (e.g., Book Club), click the New Group

    button New Group on the Address Book screen.

2. Enter the Group Name.

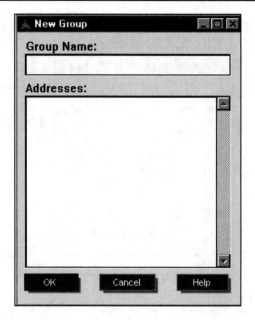

3. Enter the full e-mail addresses of each person in the group. Press Enter after typing each address.

4. Click [OK] when done.

Delete an Address Book entry

1. Click <u>M</u>ail Center, <u>A</u>ddress Book to open the Address Book.

2. Select the name to delete.

3. Click the Delete button [Delete].

4. Click Yes to confirm the deletion.

5. Click **X** in the upper right-hand corner to close the Address Book.

America Online E-mail: 18

◆ Add Attachments to a Message
◆ Open an E-Mail Attachment

Add Attachments to a Message

■ Any type of file can be sent as an attachment to an e-mail message—including text files, graphics, spreadsheets, and HTML documents.

To attach files to a message:

1. Compose the message to be sent. (See **Compose New Message** on page 87.)

2. Click the Attachments button `Attachments` at the bottom of the Write Mail screen.

3. Click the Attach button `Attach`.

4. Select the drive and folder where the file you wish to attach is located.

5. Double-click the file to attach from the Attach File dialog box.

   ✔ *Multiple files can be sent by repeating the steps above. After you have selected the multiple attachments that will accompany the e-mail message, AOL will automatically combine these files into one compressed file called a zip file. If the recipient is not using AOL 4, he or she will need a file decompression program such as PKZIP or WINZIP to open the file.*

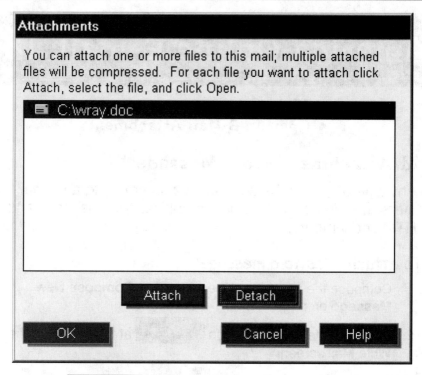

6. Click **OK**.

  ✔ *The attachment will appear at the bottom of the Write Mail screen next to the Attachments button.*

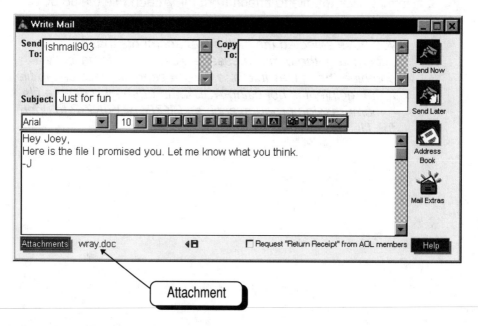

Attachment

7. If you are online, click the Send button to send the message immediately, or click the Send Later button to store the message in your Outgoing Mail if you are working offline.

Open an E-mail Attachment

- An e-mail message that arrives with a file attachment is displayed in your new mail list with a small diskette icon under the message icon.

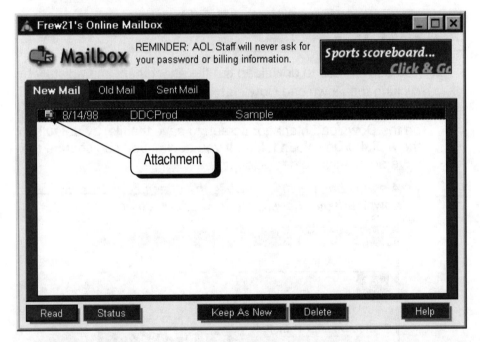

- Opening the message and viewing the attachment are two separate steps:
  1. Open the message by double-clicking on it from the New Mail list. The message will display.

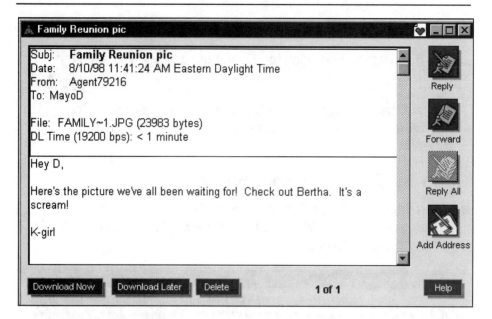

2. You can choose to download the file attachment immediately by clicking the Download Now button [Download Now] at the bottom of the displayed message screen. Click the Save button [Save] on the Download Manager screen to save the file, by default, to the AOL4.0/Download folder. If you desire, you can change the save destination folder (see page 99).

  ✔ *A status box will display while the attachment is being downloaded or transferred to your computer.*

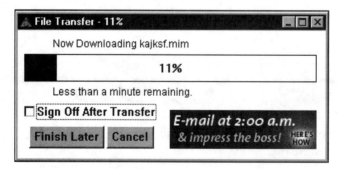

  ✔ *Click the Sign Off After Transfer checkbox if you want AOL to disconnect automatically when the transfer is complete.*

3. At the end of the download, the file transfer box will close and you will get a message confirming that the file has been transferred. Click [OK].

OR

You may choose to download the file later. Click the Download Later button Download Later to store the message in the Download Manager. When you are ready to download the file, click My Files, Download Manager, and then select the file to download. You must be online.

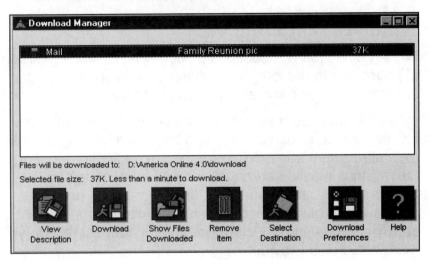

To change the default location of where files are stored:

1. Click the My Files button My Files from the AOL toolbar.
2. Click Download Manager and then the Select Destination button Select Destination from the Download Manager screen.
3. Select the desired destination from the Select Path dialog box.

   ✔ *All files will be automatically downloaded to this location.*

Search Engines: 19

Surfing vs. Searching

- The Web has many thousands of locations, containing millions of pages of information. Unfortunately, the Internet has no uniform way of tracking and indexing everything.

- Initially, it may seem easy to do research on the Web—you just connect to a relevant site and then start clicking on links to related sites. This random method of finding information on the Internet is called *surfing*. It may be interesting and fun, but there are drawbacks. Surfing is time consuming and the results are frequently inconsistent and incomplete. It can also be expensive if you are charged fees for connect time to your Internet Service Provider.

- *Searching* is a more systematic and organized way of looking for information. You can connect to one of several search sites that use *search engines* to track, catalog, and index information on the Internet.

Search Sites

- A *search site* builds its catalog using a search engine. A search engine is a software program that goes out on the Web, seeks Web sites, and catalogs them, usually by downloading their home pages.

- Search sites are classified by the way they use search engines to gather Web site data. Below and on the following page is an explanation of how the major search services assemble and index information.

Search Engines

- Search engines are sometimes called *spiders* or *crawlers* because they crawl the Web.

- Search engines constantly visit sites on the Web to create catalogs of Web pages and keep them up to date.

- Major search engines include: AltaVista, HotBot, and Open Text.

Directories

- Search *directories* are created by people who catalog information by building hierarchical indexes. Directories may be better organized than search engine sites, but may not be as complete or up-to-date as search engines that constantly check for new material on the Internet.

- Yahoo!, the oldest search service on the World Wide Web, is the best example of an Internet search directory. Other major search directories are: Infoseek, Magellan, and Lycos.

Multi-Threaded Search Engines

- Another type of search engine, called a *multi-threaded* search engine, searches other Web search sites and gathers the results of these searches for your use.

- Because they search the catalogs of other search sites, multi-threaded search sites do not maintain their own catalogs. These search sites provide more search options than subject-and-keyword search sites, and they typically return more specific information with further precision. However, multi-threaded search sites are much slower to return search results than subject-and-keyword search sites.

- Multi-threaded search sites include SavvySearch and Internet Sleuth.

■ If you are using Internet Explorer or Netscape Navigator, you can click on the Search button on the toolbar to access a number of search services.

Search Basics

- When you connect to a search site, the home page has a text box for typing the words you want to use in your search. These words are called a *text string*. The text string may be a single word or phrase.

- Once you have entered a text string, initiate the search by either pressing the Enter key or by clicking on the search button. This button may be called Search, Go Get It, Seek Now, Find, or something similar.

- For the best search results:

  - Always check for misspelled words and typing errors.

  - Use descriptive words and phrases.

  - Use synonyms and variations of words.

  - Find and follow the instructions that the search site suggests for constructing a good search.

  - Eliminate unnecessary words (the, a, an, etc.) from the search string. Concentrate on key words and phrases.

  - Test your search string on several different search sites. Search results from different sites can vary greatly.

  - Explore some of the sites that appear on your initial search and locate terms that would help you refine your search string.

Search Engines: 20

◆ Simple Searches ◆ Refine a Search ◆ Get Help

Simple Searches

■ Searches can be simple or complex, depending on how you design the search string in the text box.

■ A *simple search* uses a text string to search for matches in a search engine's catalog. A simple search is the broadest kind of search.

- The text string may be specific, such as *Social Security*, *current stock quotes*, or *Macintosh computers*, or it may be general, such as *software*, *economy*, or *computer*.

- The catalog search will return a list, typically quite large, of Web pages and URLs whose descriptions contain the text string you want to find. Frequently these searches will yield results with completely unrelated items.

■ When you start a search, the Web site searches its catalog for occurrences of your text string. The results of the search are displayed in the window of your browser.

■ Each search site has its own criteria for rating the matches of a catalog search and setting the order in which they are displayed.

■ The catalog usually searches for matches of the text string in the URLs of Web sites. It also searches for key words, phrases, and meta-tags (key words that are part of the Web page, but are not displayed in a browser) in the cataloged Web pages.

■ The information displayed on the results page will vary, depending on the search site and the search and display options you select. The most likely matches for your text string appear first in the results list, followed by other likely matches on successive pages.

✔ *There may be thousands of matches that contain your text string. The matches are displayed a page at a time. You can view the next page by clicking on the "next page" link provided at the bottom of each search results page.*

■ You can scan the displayed results to see if a site contains the information you want. Site names are clickable links. After visiting a site, you can return to the search site by clicking the Back button on your browser. You can then choose a different site to visit or perform another search.

Refine a Search

■ Suppose that you only want to view links that deal with Greek tragedies. Note, in the example below, the number of documents that were found when *Greek tragedies* was entered in this search. Since the search string didn't include a special *operator* to tell the search engine to look for sites that contain both Greek *and* tragedies, the results display sites that contain Greek *or* tragedies in addition to sites that contain Greek *and* tragedies.

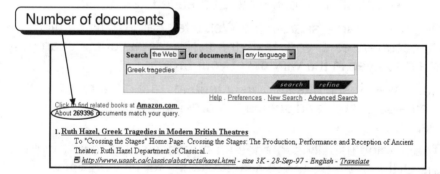

■ To reduce the number of documents in this search, use operators—words or symbols that modify the text string instead of being part of it. Enter *Greek,* space once, then enter a plus sign (+) and the word *tragedies* (Greek +tragedies) then click Search. This tells AltaVista to look for articles that contain Greek *and* tragedies in the documents. Note the results that display when the plus is added to the search.

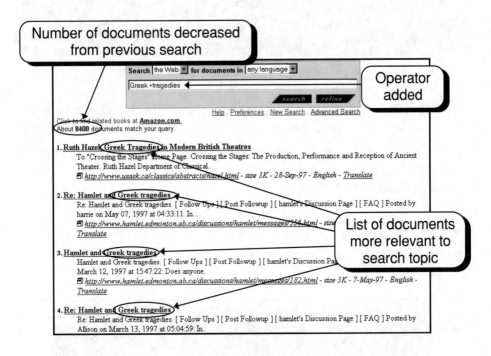

- The number of results is dramatically reduced, and the documents displayed display information that is more closely related to the topic, *Greek tragedies*.

- You can also *exclude* words by using the minus sign (-) to refine a search further and eliminate unwanted documents in the results. For example, if you wanted to find articles about Greek tragedies but not ones that deal with Hamlet, enter a search string like this: *Greek +tragedies -Hamlet*.

Get Help

- Check the Help features on the search tool that you are using to see what operators are available. Since there are no standards governing the use of operators, search sites can develop their own.

Search Engines: 21

◆ AltaVista ◆ Yahoo! ◆ excite

- Web searches can be frustrating. There are, however, a few basic tips that will almost always help you find what you want.
- Following are search tips for three of the most popular search sites. Each search site is different but some search techniques are universal.

AltaVista

http://altavista.digital.com/

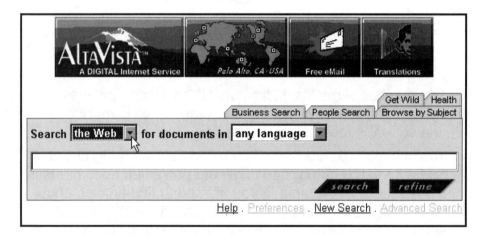

- Enter your text string in the Search box. Make sure all words are spelled correctly.
- You may modify your search string with operators to narrow the search results. This will help you find more information specifically relevant to your search.

  - To modify your search string, put a (+) in front of the words that *must* be in your results and a (–) in front of the words that must *not* be in your results.

- Always use lowercase letters when searching the Web using AltaVista unless you are using proper nouns.

- You can also enter exact phrases into the search text box. If you are looking for pages that contain an exact phrase, enclose the phrase in the Search box with quotation marks.

- Search Usenets (Newsgroups) to read public opinion and postings on thousands of topics.

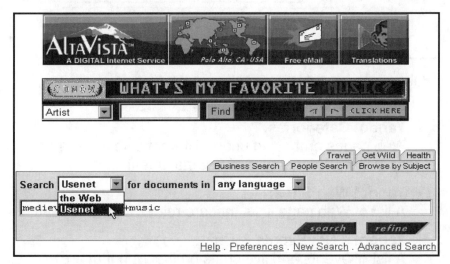

- Go to the AltaVista search areas found at the top of the search box to search a collection of Web pages and sites on everything from Travel to People.

- Click on AltaVista *Help* to get more information on searches.

Yahoo!

http://www.Yahoo.com

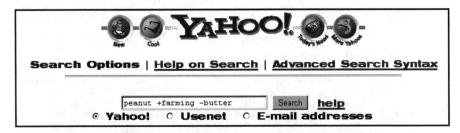

- Yahoo! searches for information in the four databases contained in its search catalog:

  - **Yahoo! Categories:**
    Web pages organized under different categories such as History, Economy, and Entertainment.

  - **Yahoo! Web Sites:**
    A list of Web page links that are relevant to your search.

  - **Yahoo!'s Net Events & Chat:**
    A list of events and live chats on the Web that are relevant based on words in your search string.

  - **Most Recent News Articles:**
    A database of over 300 online publications for articles that contain your keywords.

- Enter the keywords of your search in the search box. Make sure the words are spelled correctly.

- Be as specific as possible when entering keywords into the search box.

- Use a **(+)** in front of any keyword that must appear in the document and a **(-)** in front of words that should not.

- Yahoo! provides search syntax options to help you modify your search.

- To display search syntax options, click the *options* link next to the Search button from the home page. The following dialog box displays:

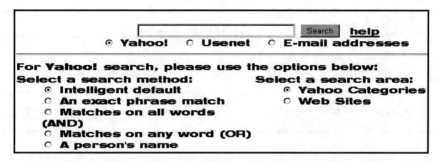

- You can also do a search by document title and URL.
- Place a *t:* in front of one or more keywords to yield Web pages with the keywords in the title of the page.
- Place a *u:* in front of keywords to yield returns with the keyword in the URL. Your search should return pages dedicated to the subject of your keywords.
- Yahoo! has specialized search areas. Click on any of the links on the Yahoo! home page to search for anything from stock quote information to buying a pet or an automobile. These links contain extensive information.

excite

http://www.excite.com/

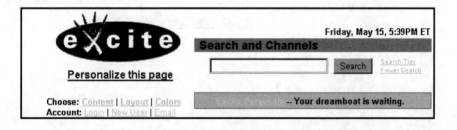

- excite searches the Web by concept using Intelligent Concept Extraction (ICE) to find the relationships between words and ideas.
- Enter concepts and ideas rather than keywords into the search box.
- You can further modify your search by adding words supplied by excite based on the keywords or phrase you've entered.

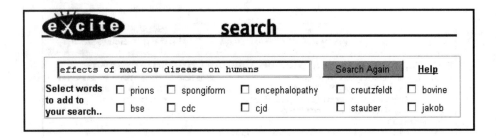

- Modify the words in your search phrase by using the (+) and (−) signs.

- Click *Help* to read more on excite search.

- You can activate a Power Search. This search uses the excite Search Wizard to help focus your search.

- Click the *Power Search* link located to the left of the search box on the excite home page. Enter the keywords or idea into the search box, as shown below.

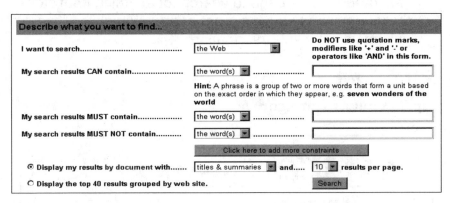

WEB RESOURCES

General Medical Resources

◆ Healthfinder ◆ Mayo Health Oasis ◆ Ask Dr. Weil
◆ Other Sites

The number of general medical advice and resource sites is growing rapidly. The information in these sites is getting better and more accessible. Now you can find out about nutrition, hundreds of common first-aid solutions, and much more.

Healthfinder™

http://www.healthfinder.org/default.htm

If you are looking for health info, be sure that you go to reputable sites, like the Federal Department of Health and Human Services' Healthfinder.

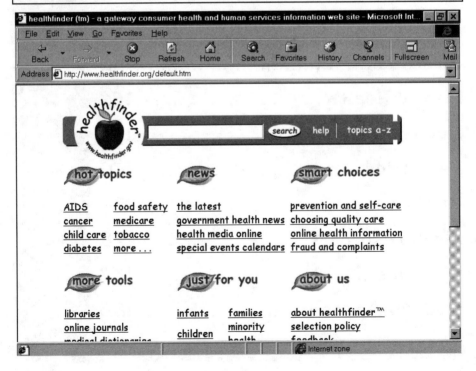

- Search by subject using the Healthfinder site. Topics include everything from the ordinary—such as the common cold—to the more obscure—such as the rare inherited vision disorder achromatopsia. Each topic links to a catalog of additional links, medical journals, support groups, and government agencies.

- The site also features excellent hot topics that cover a variety of issues such as Medicare policies, food safety, and Alzheimer's disease.

- The Healthfinder site is easy to navigate, full of important information, and interesting to explore. And, most importantly, you don't need to be a health care professional to understand the information on these pages.

Mayo Health Oasis

http://www.mayohealth.org

 Health, nutrition, and simple cures for ailments—it's all here at the Mayo Health Oasis. Click the many links to different medical areas for valuable, free medical information.

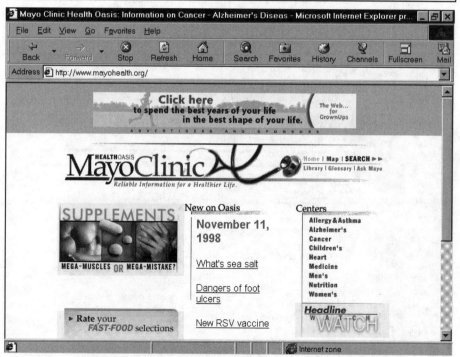

- The Mayo Health Oasis reflects the overall excellence you would expect from the highly esteemed Mayo Clinic. This easy-to-navigate site provides simple answers to a wide range of medical questions—from easy to complex. Furthermore, the information is presented in a casual, conversational tone.

- The site has information on everything from advances in cancer research to health and nutrition to women's health.

- Each Resource Center topic includes links to several other pages. Click *Ask the Mayo Physician* for answers by Mayo Clinic physicians to questions sent in by anyone with a computer and an inquiry.

- The Mayo Health Oasis has its own Newsstand and Library for reading articles and researching a variety of health topics. Click *What's Hot* for information on new medical topics that affect our daily lives.

Ask Dr. Weil

http://www.drweil.com

 If you want to learn about healthy living or find the answer to a simple health-related question, this is good place to explore.

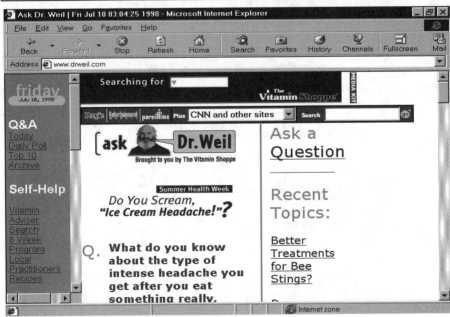

■ Even if you don't have a health concern, exploring Dr. Weil's site can be informative and entertaining. The core of the site is Dr. Weil's responses to questions that are posted by visitors to the site.

■ Go to the site to post a question or browse the archives.

■ Most of the questions address common concerns like the best way to treat a sunburn or quick cures for a stomachache. If you are looking for data on a more serious ailment, you may want to try one of the other medical sites.

■ Dr. Weil is an advocate of staying healthy through diet and exercise. He also supports trying natural remedies over strong prescription drugs.

■ The information on the page, especially under the Self-Help heading, may seem a bit New Age. But it is all sound information. And if you like to cook, be sure to check out the healthy recipes.

Other Sites

Medscape®

http://www.medscape.com

• Register for free at this site for a wealth of in-depth information. Though a lot of the material is for the health care professional, the amount of information for the layman (including a great medical dictionary) is excellent.

MSNBC Health Pages

http://www.msnbc.com/news/health_front.asp

• For current news on allergies, diet, nutrition, and all fronts of health care, visit this news giant's health pages.

Allergies

For many people, the mere mention of the word "rose" or "cat" makes them sneeze. Millions of allergy sufferers out there know that there are no easy cures, but there are lots of ways to appease the symptoms. Hundreds of Web sites offer information, remedies, and healthful advice. Misery loves company, so sniffle with other allergy sufferers online.

AllerDays®

http://www.allerdays.com

Go to this site to find the causes of allergies, pollen reports, the latest on allergy therapy and medications, and a forum where allergy sufferers share their horror and relief stories.

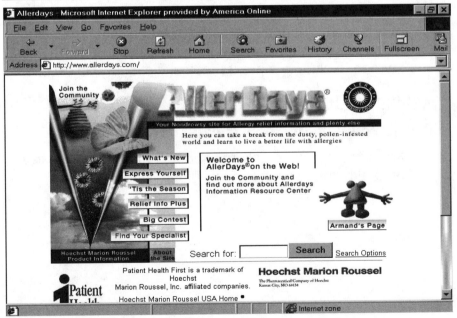

- When that nagging cold that you've had for months won't go away, visit the AllerDays site—your cold may be an allergy. This site details some telltale signs to distinguish a cold from an allergy. You can also read advice on ways to make the symptoms go away.

- Some of the allergy-relieving features of this site include a searchable database of allergy specialists and an entire area devoted to "Why we sneeze and what we can do about it."

- When the specialist can't stop you from sneezing and over-the-counter or prescription medicines aren't working, try some visual relief. Click on the *Express Yourself* link to view allergy-inspired art and read what others are sniffling about.

Allergy, Asthma & Immunology Online
http://allergy.mcg.edu

This site provides allergy sufferers with solutions through education, public advocacy groups, and research.

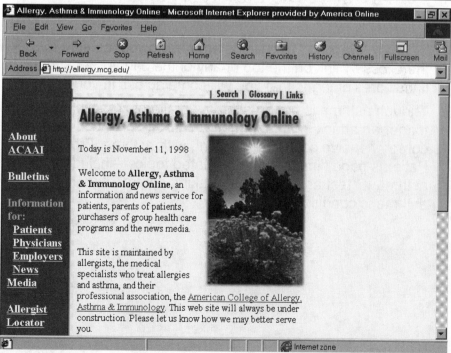

- From the home page, click on *Patients* for tons of easy-to-understand basics for allergy victims. Here you'll find a feature called *Ask Dr. Ira!* that includes allergy FAQs (frequently asked questions) and answers. A sample listing of questions follows:

- What is an allergy?
- What causes an allergic reaction?
- Who develops allergies?
- Why do people get allergies?
- What is the best method of testing for allergies?
- Do allergy shots have side effects?
- Can young children be tested?
- Is chlorine allergy common?
- Is tobacco smoke an allergen?
- Are there "non-allergic" dogs?

- If allergy terms and conditions are new to you, be sure to click the *Glossary* link on the top of any of the pages. Here you can find scores of terms that you will come across in your travels.

- Though asthma is not an allergy, an allergic reaction can trigger an attack in an asthmatic. This site provides comprehensive coverage on living with asthma. From the Patients page, link to asthma-related topics—including an asthma IQ test and a guide for taking control of your asthmatic condition.

American Academy of Allergy, Asthma & Immunology Online

http://www.aaaai.org

Since 1943, these advocates have been fighting the plight of allergy sufferers with education and research. If you are looking for relief online, visit this fact-filled site.

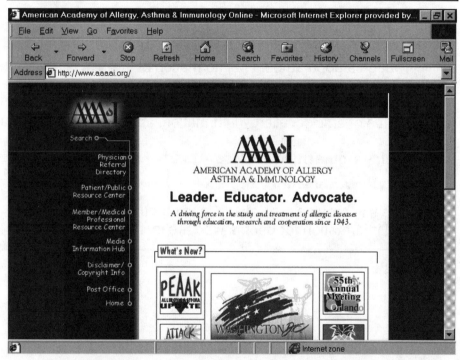

- To get started at this site, click the *Patient/Public Resource Center* on the home page. From here you can register to receive free educational bulletins, read up on allergy and asthma facts, learn about famous people with allergies and asthma (for reassurance that you're not alone), and much more. The Patient/Public page also has an area just for kids.

- This site also maintains an extensive database of physicians, which you can search by location, name, or specialty.

Other Sites

The Food Allergy Network
http://www.foodallergy.org

- FAN is a nonprofit organization that provides information and support for people living with food-related allergies. This site features research, food updates, and general information about food allergies.

Doctor's Guide to Allergies Information & Resources
http://www.pslgroup.com/allergies.htm

- Though a good amount of information at this site is aimed at health care professionals, allergy sufferers are bound to find something of interest at this comprehensive site with scores of articles, allergy information, and excellent links.

Non-Dairy Something to Moo About
http://www.non-dairy.org

- This site provides recipes, shopping guidelines, research, and information for people who are lactose-intolerant.

Alternative Medicine

◆ Alternative Medicine Online
◆ Alternative Health News ◆ Other Sites

Alternative medicine has its roots in Eastern medical therapies. More and more, holistic approaches are merging with conventional Western medicine for more effective treatments of illness.

Alternative Medicine Online

http://library.advanced.org/24206

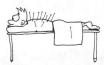 If you want to learn more about alternative medicine, its origins, and various medical therapies available, this site is a terrific resource.

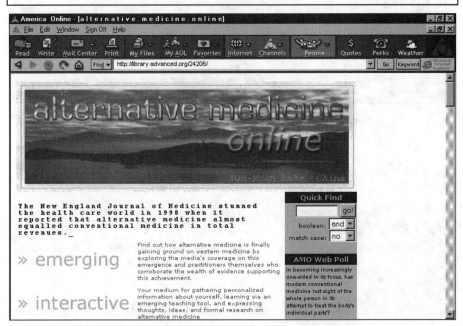

- The main focus of this site is to dispel misconceptions about alternative medicine. Take the Myth or Fact quiz to learn about how alternative medicine and alternative medical therapies differ from Western treatments and philosophies.

- Read about dozens of common alternative medicine therapies and holistic models of health care. Or, click the *Facts & Stats* link to learn more about the rising popularity of holistic medicine.

- Through the interactive area you can communicate with others via the Alternative Medicine Online bulletin board or the online chats.

Alternative Health News

http://www.altmedicine.com

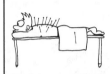 This award-winning site strives to keep the Internet community informed with links to credible media sources and experts in the field of alternative medicine.

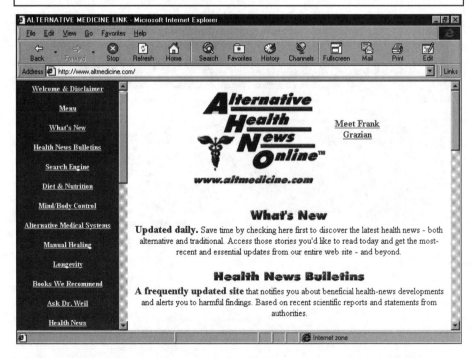

- Go to the What's New area for the most current studies in alternative medicine. The Health News Bulletin posts new health and medical developments, preventative measures, and alternative approaches.

- Take the Nutrition quiz to develop a profile based on your height, weight, and body frame. Learn about the healing properties of different vitamins, understand the positive effects of a macrobiotic diet, read news about nutrition research, and get tips on herbal remedies.
- If you want to find a qualified holistic specialist in your area, consult the local practitioners database for more information.

Other Sites

The Alternative Medicine Home Page

http://www.pitt.edu/~cbw/altm.html

- The University of Pittsburgh's alternative medicine site offers links to related Web sites, newsgroups and mailing lists, and government resources.

National Center for Complementary and Alternative Medicine

http://altmed.od.nih.gov/nccam

- If you have questions about alternative medical therapies, medicines, or practices, visit this site. This organization falls under the mandate of the National Institute of Health.

Countway Web Resources

http://www.countway.med.harvard.edu/countway/webref/altmed.html

- Find links to sites with valuable information on acupuncture, herbal medicine, mind-body medicine, as well as associations and organizations that deal with alternative medicine.

ALTERNATIVE

123

Arthritis

◆ Arthritis Foundation ◆ ArthritisNet
◆ National Institute of Arthritis and Musculoskeletal
and Skin Diseases (NIAMS)
◆ Other Sites

Arthritis afflicts nearly one in every six people in the United States alone, including children. The good news is that in most cases this often-crippling disease can be controlled with early detection, medication, proper diet, and exercise.

Arthritis Foundation

http://www.arthritis.org

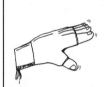

The Arthritis Foundation has been a leader in arthritis research and treatment for over 50 years. Here you can find medical literature, nationwide support groups, and valuable lifestyle tips for people living with arthritis.

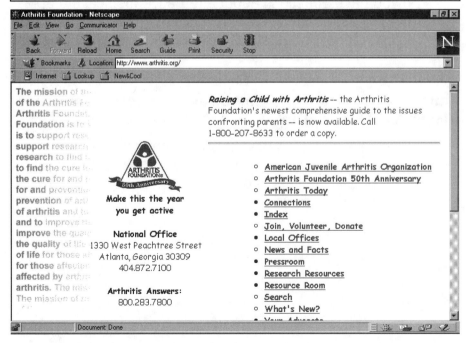

The mission of the Arthritis Foundation is to support research to find the cure for and prevention of arthritis and to improve the quality of life for those affected by arthritis. The mission of the

Raising a Child with Arthritis -- the Arthritis Foundation's newest comprehensive guide to the issues confronting parents -- is now available. Call 1-800-207-8633 to order a copy.

Make this the year you get active

National Office
1330 West Peachtree Street
Atlanta, Georgia 30309
404.872.7100

Arthritis Answers:
800.283.7800

○ American Juvenile Arthritis Organization
○ Arthritis Foundation 50th Anniversary
○ Arthritis Today
● Connections
● Index
○ Join, Volunteer, Donate
● Local Offices
○ News and Facts
● Pressroom
● Research Resources
● Resource Room
○ Search
○ What's New?

- Among the great things found on this site are the *Tip* links that connect to single-topic pages where you can read up on everything from carpal tunnel syndrome in the workplace to soaking in a hot tub to relieve arthritis pain. Each link includes helpful tips and possible preventative measures.

- The Resource Room offers both online and offline materials geared to helping you or someone you care about cope with arthritis. Read about managing arthritis, how to purchase books and educational brochures, and information about local services and programs.

- Six times a year the Arthritis Foundation publishes *Arthritis Today*. The recipient of over 107 awards, *Arthritis Today* includes practical tips submitted by readers, the latest cutting-edge research and technologies, and helpful hints on proper exercise and nutrition. Read excerpts from the magazine online.

- Check this site for listings for local chapters of the Arthritis Foundation throughout the U.S. and special programs for children, parents, and teachers.

ArthritisNet

http://www.arthritisnet.com

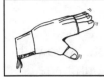 This site tempers the seriousness of expert information about arthritis with a sense of humor.

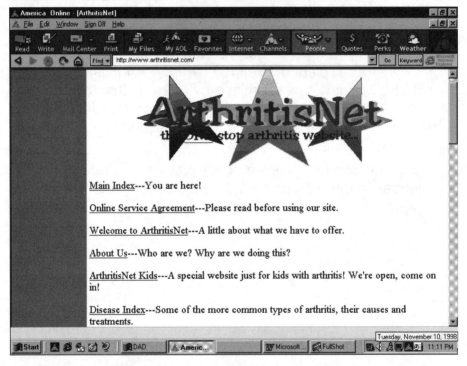

- What makes ArthritisNet so personable is the amount of Internet visitor input. You'll find a lot of information submitted by people living with arthritis.

- For "news, laughs, tips and more" go to the News area and subscribe to the free ArthritisNet newsletter. Experts in the fields of fitness, pharmaceuticals, and arthritis medicine contribute articles to this weekly online publication.

- The ArthritisNet Chatroom is up and running 24 hours a day with hosted chats scheduled four times a week on arthritis-related topics. Be sure to read "Ask Annie," the ArthritisNet Dear Abby. Each week she answers new questions submitted by visitors to the site.

- You can also order practical supplies such as books, canes, orthopedic supplies, as well as alternative therapies such as herbal remedies and aromatherapy products.

National Institute of Arthritis and Musculoskeletal and Skin Diseases (NIAMS)

http://www.nih.gov/niams/

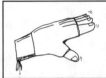 Part of the National Institutes of Health (NIH), NIAMS leads the federal effort on research into the causes, treatment, and prevention of arthritis and musculoskeletal and skin diseases.

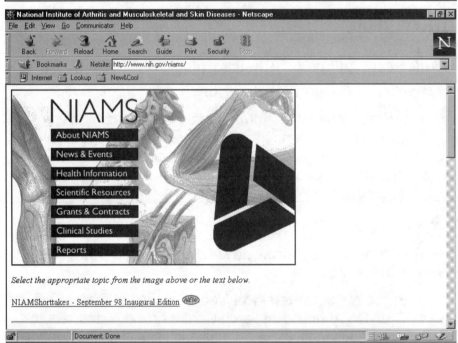

- Although this site presents much of the information in scientific or medical terms, you'll find plenty of easy-to-understand information on the research and treatments of such conditions as osteoarthritis, polymyositis, and rheumatoid arthritis.

- Read the Q&A areas for simple explanations to frequently asked questions about arthritis and explanations of advances in treatments.
- Stressing the importance of exercise as a way to combat the effects of arthritis, NIAMS offers tips on how to begin and maintain an exercise regimen with the support of your physician.
- For more in-depth information on medical advances and treatment, go the *Reports* link found on the home page. There you will find links to reports on different scientific workshops and symposiums that discuss arthritis research and clinical applications.

Other Sites

American College Of Rheumatology

http://www.rheumatology.org

- While much of the information on this site can only be accessed by members of the American College of Rheumatology, nonmembers can access useful patient information. Click the *Rheumatology* link for a gateway to dozens of top Web sites.

Thurston Arthritis Research Center

http://www.med.unc.edu/wrkunits/3ctrpgm/ mac/welcome.htm

- Based at the University of North Carolina at Chapel Hill, the Thurston Arthritis Research Center provides answers to many questions about arthritis and links to online support groups and other Web sites. Visit Cafe Thurston by clicking the *Do You Have Arthritis?* link from the home page.

Cancer

◆ American Cancer Society ◆ CancerNet
◆ Other Sites

Although consulting medical sites on the Web should never replace a private consultation with a qualified physician, you can use Web resources to learn more about cancer treatments, research, and support organizations.

American Cancer Society

http://www.cancer.org

 This 85-year-old organization is one of the great pioneers of cancer research and public advocacy.

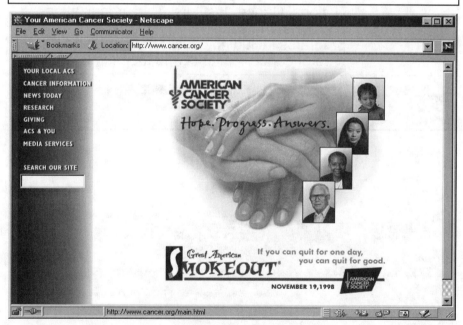

- The American Cancer Society is unparalleled in its efforts to provide responsible, expert information on all types of cancer. Find information on common cancers such as breast, prostate, and lung cancers, as well as rarer cancers like esophageal cancer and Hodgkin's disease.

129

- Along with definitions of specific diseases, you will find information on how to detect cancer, risk factors, questions to ask your physicians, and treatments for each cancer type. If you have any questions, the ACS provides a toll-free number where you can call for more information.
- You can also order free American Cancer Society publications online. Search their database by cancer type for books and brochures dealing with specific topics.
- For a look at hundreds of cancer-related issues, visit *News Today*. There you can read top news stories, articles written on medical, insurance, and political issues, and reports on new breakthroughs in cancer research.

CancerNet

http://cancernet.nci.nih.gov

CancerNet is the Web site sponsored by the National Cancer Institute. This organization conducts and supports a wide range of programs including cancer research and the care of cancer patients and their families.

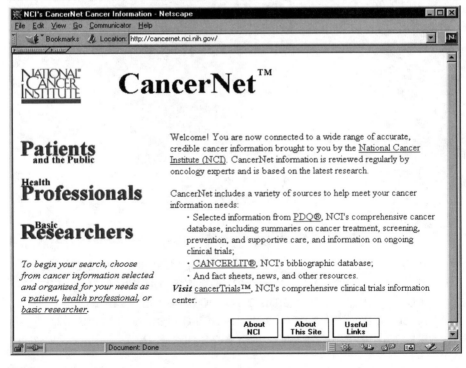

- This site features information on many different types of cancer, as well as descriptions and explanations of screening procedures, prevention, and treatments. The material is comprehensive, concise, and easy to understand. A good portion of this material is also available in Spanish.

- An extensive database on the procedures of clinical trials, including answers to questions you may have if you are thinking of participating in a trial, is available at this site. Clinical trials are necessary in the process of developing and evaluating new drug therapies, treatments, and preventative measures.

- Click on the *Supportive Care* link from the home page for more information about support groups for those with cancer and the people who live with them.

- You can also link to other organizations and areas within the National Cancer Institute. CancerLit®, for instance, is NCI's bibliographic database, containing cancer-related literature gathered over the last thirty years.

- The Kid's Home Page offers links to Web sites specifically geared to young people with cancer, as well as activities and stories for children with cancer.

C
A
N
C
E
R

Other Sites

National Coalition For Cancer Survivorship
http://www.cansearch.org

- As it says on their home page, NCCS is "a grassroots network of individuals and organizations working on behalf of people with all types of cancer."

National Childhood Cancer Foundation
http://www.nccf.org

- This organization supports pediatric treatments and research projects at over 115 pediatric institutions. Find links to Web resources, inspiring stories of children surviving cancer, and information on what you can do to promote and support pediatric cancer research.

OncoLink®
http://oncolink.upenn.edu

- This educational site—the Web site for the University of Pennsylvania Cancer Center—offers help for people coping with cancer, book reviews, and news on the latest breakthrough treatments.

Dentistry

◆ ADA® Online™ ◆ Dental ResourceNet
◆ Dr. Spieler's Dental Zone ◆ Other Sites

Keeping a healthy smile takes lots of brushing, flossing, and trips to the dentist. When it comes to your teeth, a little preventative maintenance will keep your choppers sparkling for years to come.

ADA® Online™

http://www.ada.org

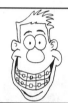

The American Dental Association (ADA), founded in 1859, has brought its dedication to teeth, gums, and oral hygiene online. Visit this site to learn about all aspects of dental care.

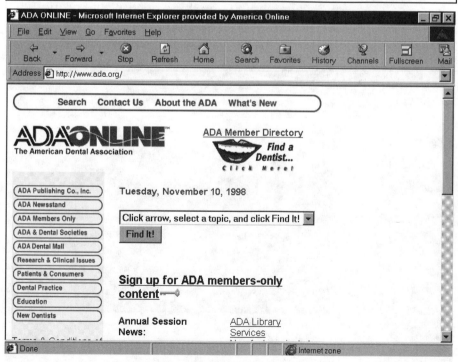

- This site covers it all—from information on baby bottle tooth decay to the latest studies on the pros and cons of having your teeth bleached.

- If you are in the market for a new dentist or a specialist, search ADA's database of dentists. The database can be searched by city. Indicate if you are looking for a specialist.

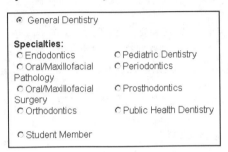

```
⊙ General Dentistry

Specialties:
  ○ Endodontics              ○ Pediatric Dentistry
  ○ Oral/Maxillofacial       ○ Periodontics
  Pathology
  ○ Oral/Maxillofacial       ○ Prosthodontics
  Surgery
  ○ Orthodontics             ○ Public Health Dentistry

  ○ Student Member
```

Dental ResourceNet

http://www.dentalcare.com

Procter & Gamble's dental care site answers questions about everything essential to proper dental care and dental procedures.

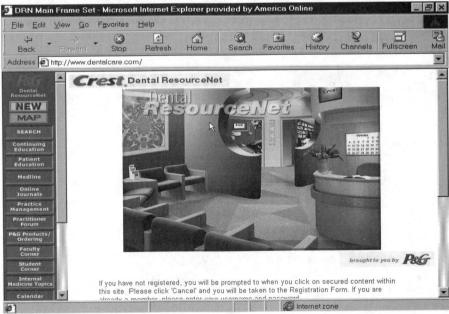

- The Procter & Gamble Crest Dental ResourceNet answers the most common questions about effective dental care. Although many areas on this site are primarily for the use of health care professionals who must register to access this information, there are many informative areas that are available to laymen.

- Although going to the dentist can be a frightening proposition, this site makes the most out of what may at first seem unappealing. Click on the *Patient Education* link to learn more about such topics as proper dental hygiene, wisdom tooth treatments, and root canals.

- Click on the *Consumer Site* link to go to the P&G House Call area. Here you can find links to dental care for adults and seniors. Learn how osteoporosis and menopause affect your mouth, compare the benefits of dentures versus implants, read about high blood pressure concerns, and much more.

Dr. Spieler's Dental Zone

http://www.saveyoursmile.com

Dr. Spieler is a teeth fan, and his mission is to make sure that "your smile lasts a lifetime."

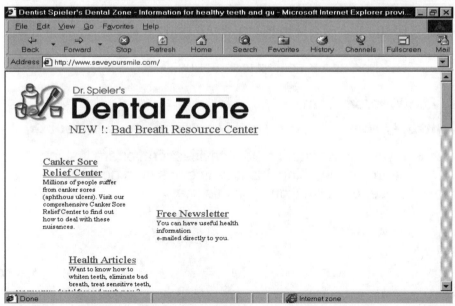

- Dr. Spieler's mission is to reassure people that yes, you do need to take proper care of your teeth, but no, dental hygiene and going to the dentist do not have to be unpleasant. It's just a matter of a little preventative care and a dentist you trust.

- The home page of this site is not overly cluttered with links, making the site easy to navigate. Some of the options on the home page include a link to register for Dr. Spieler's free newsletter, which is e-mailed to subscribers once a month. Also included is a link to *Health Articles*, which features information and advice on what to do about sensitive teeth, how to conquer your phobia of going to the dentist, teeth whitening, and more.

- An excellent feature of the site is an area dedicated to parents' concerns with their children's teeth. From the parents' pages learn about getting your children to establish good brushing habits and what to do to avoid baby bottle tooth decay.

Other Sites

The Adventures of Mr. Reach

http://www.jnjoralhealth.com

- Sponsored by Johnson & Johnson, this site is extremely kid- and family-friendly. Kids can check out the "Dunk Mr. Plaque" game and learn about good dental habits, while parents can read up on proper oral development for children and teaching techniques.

The Wisdom Tooth

http://www.umanitoba.ca/outreach/wisdomtooth

- If you are wondering how cavities form or are just in search of brushing tips, flossing tips, and general oral hygiene information, visit this site.

Diabetes

◆ The American Diabetes Association
◆ The Juvenile Diabetes Foundation
◆ National Institute of Diabetes and Digestive
and Kidney Diseases ◆ Other Sites

Complications developing from diabetes comprise one of the major causes of death in the U.S. Diabetes is also a major cause of blindness and kidney disease, and it multiplies a person's risk of heart disease by 400%. There is currently no cure for diabetes, but the disease can be controlled and treated. Diabetics and their loved ones, therefore, can benefit greatly by researching this illness and learning more about their options.

The American Diabetes Association
http://www.diabetes.org

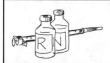 ADA's site provides valuable information for diabetics and their families, as well as for medical practitioners and those who want to volunteer or make donations.

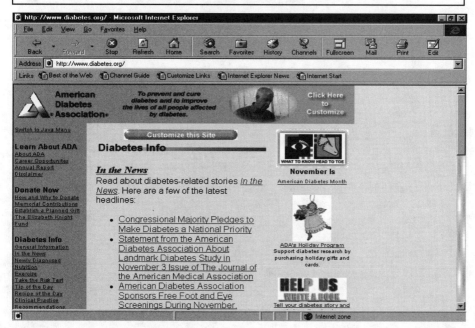

- The American Diabetes Association's mission—to prevent and cure diabetes, and to improve the lives of all people affected by diabetes—is reflected in its site. Boasting dozens of links to a wide variety of subjects and helpful topics, from *Nutrition* and *Exercise* to *Research* and *Health Insurance*, this site gives quick but thorough access to available resources.

- In order to take advantage of any up-to-the-minute medical and technological advances, diabetics and their families need to be informed. Click *In the News* for the latest diabetes-related stories from around the world. Likewise, click *Research News* for the latest scientific findings.

- Every diabetic knows that until a cure is found, proper self-management of the disease is the key to living a healthy life. Check out the Diabetes Info links for tips and recommendations on day-to-day self-care. (And don't worry, this is *fun* stuff, including delicious diabetes-friendly recipes and exercise tips.)

The Juvenile Diabetes Foundation

http://www.jdfcure.org

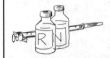 JDF's goal is to find a cure for diabetes and its complications. Check here to find out the latest on what is being done to reach that goal.

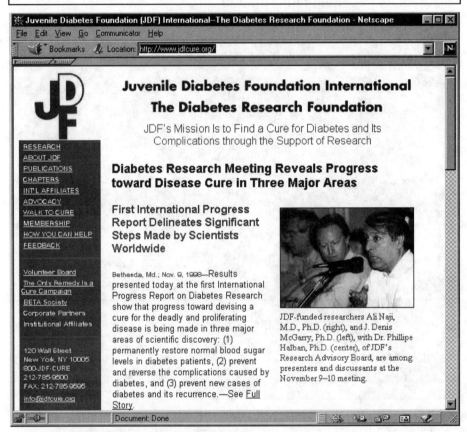

- The Juvenile Diabetes Foundation is a not-for-profit, voluntary agency that funds research to find a cure for diabetes. Check out the *About JDF* link for an overview of the Foundation—including an Introduction by Mary Tyler Moore.

- How close are we to a cure? This is the place to find out—and to help in the search. Check out the *Walk to Cure* and *How You Can Help* links to get involved.

National Institute of Diabetes and Digestive and Kidney Diseases

http://www.niddk.nih.gov

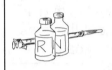 NIDDK is part of the National Institutes of Health. Their site offers a rundown of their ongoing research projects and also provides health information.

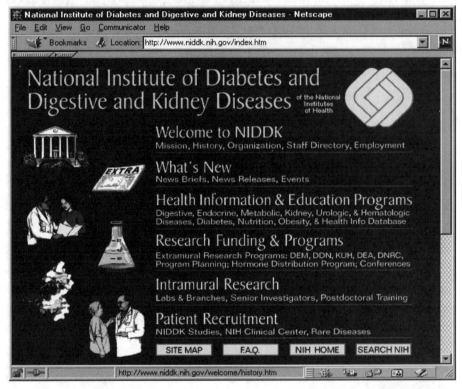

- Because NIDDK sponsors and conducts medical research, their Web site is filled with information about their latest studies and findings. Check out the *Patient Recruitment* links if you are interested in participating in any of the studies.

- Although the site is geared toward the Institute's research, you'll find plenty of health information available to diabetics. Click the *Diabetes* link under Health Information & Education Programs for an exhaustive list of diabetes-related materials and links to other programs and resources. (*Diabetes Overview* is a good place to start.)

Other Sites

Diabetes.com
http://www.diabetes.com

- Put together by professional medical writers, this site calls itself a "major gateway to diabetes information on the Internet"—and it is!

Children with Diabetes On-line Community
http://www.childrenwithdiabetes.com

- A fabulous resource for diabetic kids, their families, and adult diabetics, too.

CDC's Diabetes and Public Health Resource
http://www.cdc.gov/nccdphp/ddt

- This organization's mission is to translate scientific discovery and convert it into daily clinical practice. Their site gives a general statistical look at diabetes and the latest treatment options.

Doctors

◆ **American Medical Association Physician Select**
◆ **American Board of Medical Specialties**
Physician Locator ◆ **Other Sites**

One of the most important choices a person can make about health care is the selection of a doctor. Besides primary care doctors, many health plans permit members the freedom to select a specialist of their own choosing. Internet health consumer resources can help you find and evaluate physician credentials and locate doctors in your area.

The Doctor Directory

http://www.doctordirectory.com

The Doctor Directory boasts listings for virtually every physician practicing in the U.S.

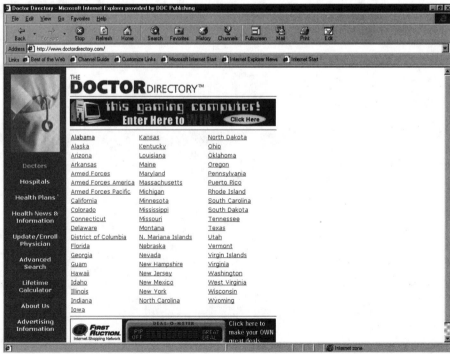

- This fast, user-friendly site offers quick access to doctors and health providers in every U.S. state as well as Guam, the Virgin Islands, and the Armed Forces. This is also a good source for health and news information and top medical stories.

- From the home page, you can easily follow links to your home town (or a city you want to research) and find a list of medical practitioners, their contact information, languages they speak, affiliated hospitals and health plans, and a map to the office.

- You can also search this award-winning site for hospitals and health plans. Use the advanced search feature to search by specialty, city, state, ZIP Code, or 5- or 10-mile radius.

American Medical Association Physician Select

http://www.ama-assn.org/aps/amahg.htm

Find important information on a doctor or specialist, such as medical school, year of graduation, residency training, address, and phone number.

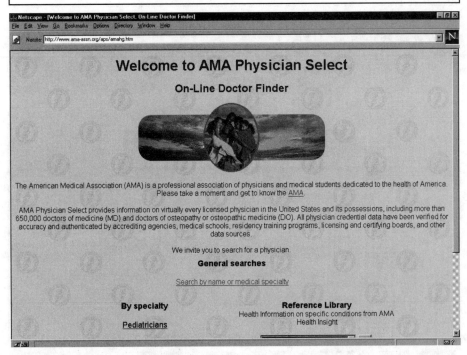

Welcome to AMA Physician Select

On-Line Doctor Finder

The American Medical Association (AMA) is a professional association of physicians and medical students dedicated to the health of America. Please take a moment and get to know the AMA.

AMA Physician Select provides information on virtually every licensed physician in the United States and its possessions, including more than 650,000 doctors of medicine (MD) and doctors of osteopathy or osteopathic medicine (DO). All physician credential data have been verified for accuracy and authenticated by accrediting agencies, medical schools, residency training programs, licensing and certifying boards, and other data sources.

We invite you to search for a physician.

General searches

Search by name or medical specialty

By specialty   Reference Library
                        Health Information on specific conditions from AMA
Pediatricians   Health Insight

- This AMA Web site is a reliable source of current and authoritative medical information. Part of the site is available only to AMA members and requires a password. However, the non-member areas are vast, comprehensive, well organized, and easily searchable, such as the On-line doctor area.
- The AMA database lists over 650,000 doctors, along with their credentials. Search the database by name or medical specialty.
- The AMA site also includes a wealth of other medical-related topics. Click a subject in the Reference Library list or click the *AMA* link for more information.

American Board of Medical Specialties Physician Locator

http://www.certifieddoctor.org/

 This site tracks the certification of over 540,000 board-certified medical specialists. You can instantly verify certification status and obtain vital details about a specialist.

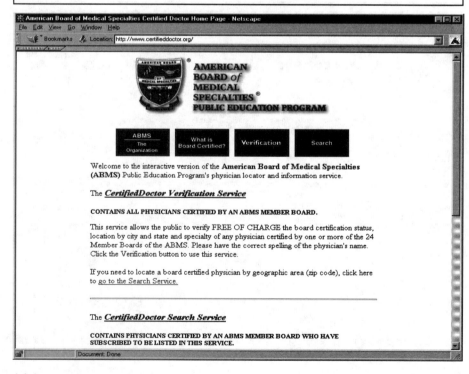

- There are twenty-four approved medical specialty boards in United States that fall under the auspices of the American Board of Medical Specialties. The ABMS maintains a list of thousands of board-certified physicians and the details of their specialization. This information is available free-of-charge to the public.

- To find out whether a physician is board-certified, click on the *CertifiedDoctor Verification Service* link and enter the doctor's name. If the doctor is certified and has subscribed to this service, your search will return a list of the doctor's telephone number, address, heath plan affiliations, and more.

- To get a listing of board-certified doctors in your area by specialty, click on the *CertifiedDoctor Search Service* link. If a doctor is not listed among your search results from the CertifiedDoctor area, it does not necessarily mean he is not a certified specialist. Doctors must subscribe to be listed in this particular area. However, all board-certified physicians are included in the CertifiedDoctor Verification database.

Other Sites

Web Health Network
http://www.whn.com/

- The WHN database includes thousands of listings for doctors, dentists, alternative practitioners, clinics, hospitals, insurance providers, and more.

Administrators in Medicine
http://www.docboard.org/

- There are fourteen participating states that will give you background on doctors including whether a doctor has been sued for malpractice in the past ten years.

American Holistic Health Association
http://ahha.org

- The AHHA site contains a searchable database to find a holistic practitioner by name or area, find resource and networking links, and information on local groups support network.

145

Eye, Ear, Nose, & Throat

◆ EyeNet ◆ National Eye Institute ◆ NIDCD
◆ Other Sites

Whether you're suffering from itchy eyes, swimmer's ear, or motion sickness, you can get a dose of preventative medicine online. Although many sites are geared toward health care practitioners, you'll find that much of the available information is easy to read, understand, and navigate. Because more and more people are turning to the Web to boost their medical IQs, you'll find that even institutions and universities have links for the general public.

EyeNet

http://www.eyenet.org

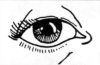 Published by the American Academy of Ophthalmology, EyeNet is an excellent resource for eye health, news, and views.

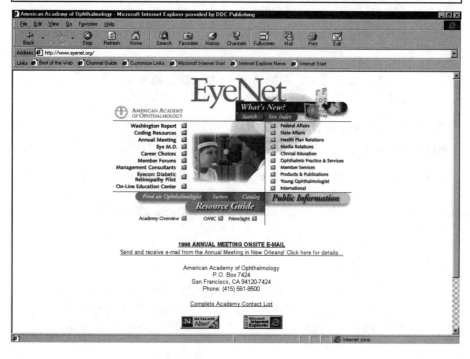

- Click the *Public Information* link for easy navigation to pages about eye conditions, diseases, anatomy, and corrective problems. You can also access public services and FAQs.

- If you're looking for an ophthalmologist for yourself or your family, you can use EyeNet's online directory to find a listing of participating doctors by name, specialty, or location.

- This attractive site also has special tips on school eye safety, numerous links to other eye care sites, and information about referral services, support groups, and other organizations.

- You can also check out their online catalog for various eye care products and services.

National Eye Institute

http://www.nei.nih.gov

 Visit the National Eye Institute's site for the latest information on eye diseases and vision research.

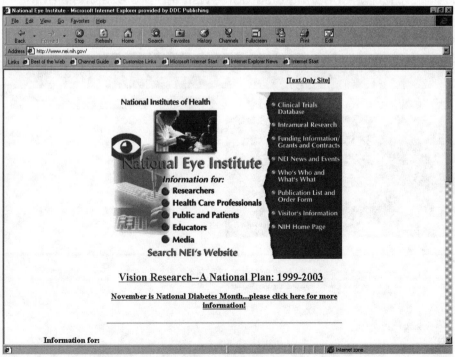

- NEI, part of the National Institutes of Health, serves doctors, researchers, educators, and laymen. Unless you're a health professional, the best place to start is the *Public and Patients* link on the home page. Find out if you're at risk for eye disease and discover sources that you can contact for aid and information.

- The NEI site includes a vast amount of information about educational programs and research news. Click the *NEI News and Events* link to learn about the latest medical discoveries, issues of concern, congressional testimonies, and clinical alerts.

- Even if you're not a health professional or educator, you may find links of interest in other areas of the NEI site. If you can't find what you're looking for, you can request information from NEI directly by using their online form.

NIDCD

http://www.nih.gov/nidcd

For answers to questions about speech and hearing disorders, visit the professionals at the National Institute on Deafness and Other Communication Disorders Web site.

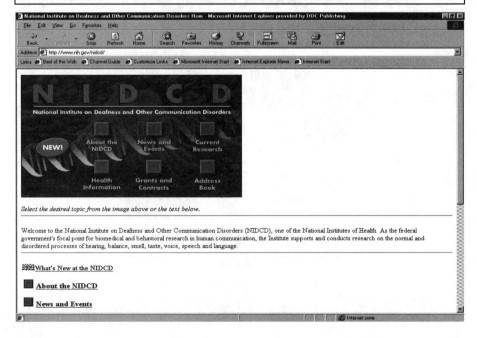

- Forty-six million Americans have disorders that affect their processes of hearing, speech, smell, taste, or language. The NIDCD has established a massive database for the sole purpose of disseminating information about these problems to the public.

- Click the *Health Information* link to access the Information Clearinghouse database, publications, resource directory links, a glossary, FAQs, and more.

- In addition to current research, news, and events links, you can access the Address Book to locate NIDCD staff, professionals, and organizations.

Other Sites

American Academy of Otolaryngology

http://www.entnet.org

- Visit the largest organization of eye, ear, nose, and throat specialists online. Learn about disorders and how to recognize them. Locate otolaryngology resources on the Internet, visit a virtual museum, and link to related discussion groups.

Ear, Nose, and Throat Information Center

http://www.netdoor.com/entinfo

- This simple yet informative public service site has numerous brochures provided by the American Academy of Otolaryngology that you can read online. Get specific facts on ear, nose, throat, and related topics.

Prevent Blindness America

http://www.preventblindness.org

- The nation's leading volunteer eye health and safety organization offers thorough information on various eye problems, eye care solutions, safety tips, news, education, and resources.

EYE, EAR, NOSE, & THROAT

Health Care Providers

◆ Employer Quality Partnership ◆ Health Pages
◆ Other Sites

As a health care consumer, it is important to know what kinds of choices are available. This means looking for a plan that suits your particular needs and doesn't break the bank. In many cases, you can choose a health care option through your employer. You can learn more about health care online and find ways to maximize your options.

Employer Quality Partnership

http://www.eqp.org/

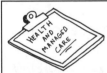 The mission of EQP is to help employers, employees, and self-employed people make more effective use of their current health plan or find a better one.

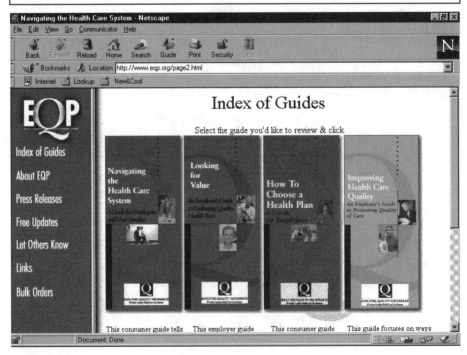

- This is one of the best sites on the Web if you really want to get a handle on understanding health care. You can choose from four downloadable guides, each with valuable information to help you understand your health care options.

- If you get health care through your place of work, read the guide for employees for advice on choosing and using a health plan. Learn how different plans work, what you should know when you see a doctor, and ways to handle coverage problems.

- Whether you're an employer, an employee, or self-employed, you'll come away from this site with a better understanding of how the health care system works, how you can influence health plans, how to evaluate the quality of medical care you're getting, and, ultimately, how to become a better health care consumer.

Health Pages

http://www.thehealthpages.com/

This site enables you to compare doctors, dentists, health plans, maternity services, and mammography clinics based on doctor credentials, cost, availability, and location.

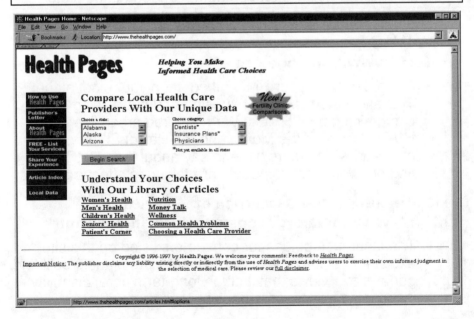

151

- One of the great features about this site is that you can search for a health care plan or search for a dentist, doctor, or clinic that accepts a specific insurance plan, and then compare your results. To begin your comparison shopping of health care plans, choose your state and make a choice from the insurance category.

- The information in the Health Pages comes from a variety of sources including federal and state government organizations and medical or professional licensing boards. The Health Pages also surveys physicians, hospitals, and health plans directly. Wherever possible, the site verifies information from multiple sources.

- For further research, review the library of articles on topics like women's health, senior health, and nutrition. Get advice on general health care information and how to choose the best provider.

Other Sites

The Blue Cross and Blue Shield Association Web Site
http://www.bluecares.com

- Health care trends and Blue Cross Blue Shield affiliates are both available within this site. Also included are a body atlas, policy alerts on both the federal and state level, and the latest advances in health care.

The HMO Page
http://www.hmopage.org

- Got a beef with your HMO? If so, then you're not alone. This site is dedicated to exposing and addressing complaints about HMOs. With featured areas like the HMO Atrocity of the Month and the Hall of Shame, you can read what others have to say about their HMOs and find out what actions people are taking to effect a change.

Health Insurance Association of America
http://www.hiaa.org/consumerinfo/index.html

- The insurance guides for consumers listed on this site explain most major insurance health care plans. You'll find general overviews that include long-term care, disability income insurance, and medical savings accounts.

Heart & Cardiovascular Disease

◆ **American Heart Association**
◆ **The Mining Company** ◆ **HeartPoint** ◆ **Other Sites**

Cardiovascular disease claims the lives of more Americans each year than the next seven leading causes of death combined. Fortunately, you can take simple steps to improve your health and decrease your risk for heart problems. Access the nation's leading health organizations online and increase your heart-smart awareness in a matter of mouse clicks.

American Heart Association®

http://www.americanheart.org

 The American Heart Association is one of the world's premier health organizations, dedicated to fighting America's number one killer.

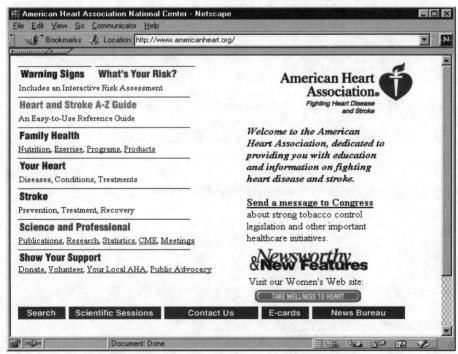

- Founded by six cardiologists in 1924, the American Heart Association has grown to more than four million volunteers nationwide. The AHA Web site is an excellent resource for facts about heart disease and stroke, preventative measures for a healthier heart, and ways to show support in your own community.

- If you're looking for specific information, you can find topics quickly in the *Heart and Stroke A–Z Guide*. Or, you can browse through the site by category to learn about risk factors, warning signs, conditions and treatments, recovery, and the latest advances in research. Get healthy-heart recipes and learn ways to improve the lifestyle of your entire family.

- The AHA also has an area devoted specifically to women's health that includes topics on self care, physicians information, public advocacy, heart and stroke education, women's forums, directories, and featured stories.

The Mining Company

http://heartdisease.miningco.com

 The guides at the Mining Company have created a comprehensive site about heart disease, complete with articles, journals, organizations, and online forums.

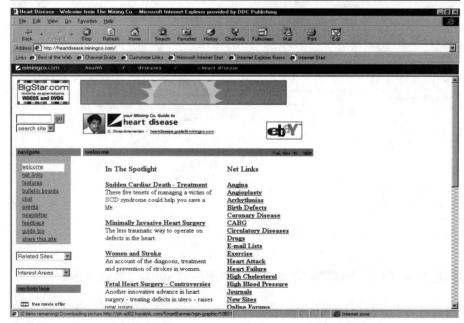

- If you're just beginning to uncover online resources, the Mining Company's site for heart disease is a great place to start. You can find everything you're looking for right on their home page, which is compiled by a cardiac surgeon.

- Click any of the Net Links on the home page to get pages of detailed links to related sites. Or, read featured articles about new treatments, medical advances, and technological breakthroughs.

- Perhaps the best feature of this site is its community aspect. You can post questions or share your concerns about heart disease on the bulletin boards, chat with the site doctor, or sign up to receive free *Healthzine* newsletters.

HeartPoint

http://www.heartpoint.com

 "Health Information You Can Trust," compiled and organized by medical professionals dedicated to providing patients with reliable resources about heart disease.

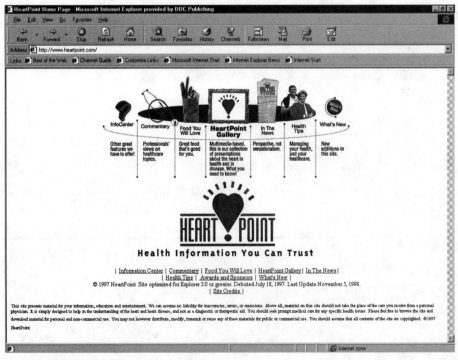

- The HeartPoint Web site has the same kind of warmth and information you might expect to find in the waiting room of your family health practitioner.

- Be sure to visit the HeartPoint Gallery, a well-designed animated presentation of various heart conditions with extensive descriptions. The site adds new cardiology topics regularly, and you can request information on specific subjects.

- Get tips to improve your health and make the most out of your health care. Read relevant news articles, find out what doctors think about medicine in society, and browse through past archives.

- You can find tasty ways to improve your health with monthly heart-smart recipes created by the site's nutritionist and culinary chef. Check for previously featured recipes in the archives.

Other Sites

Cardiology Compass

http://www.cardiologycompass.com

- Cardiology Compass is a quick navigation site with thousands of links to online cardiovascular resource centers. This site offers a no-frills, easy-to-read list of links to educational sites, professional organizations, newsgroups, e-mail addresses, cardiology guides, medical resources, online journals and publications, and nation-wide research centers.

American College of Cardiology

http://www.acc.org/login/index.taf

- You must register to access the information at this site. Registration is free, simple, and worthwhile. You'll find numerous journal articles, educational databases, exhibits, community programs, patient education features, and more.

Heart Information Network

http://www.heartinfo.org

- This site has it all: timely journal articles, nutrition guides, physician and clinic directories, a question-and-answer library, products and services, and a medical glossary.

The National Heart, Lung, and Blood Institute

http://www.nhlbi.nih.gov/nhlbi/nhlbi.htm

- This easy-to-use site offers a list of links to online resources. Find information about cardiovascular, lung, and blood disorders, publications, educational links, and research studies.

HEART DISEASE

157

Hospitals

◆ Hospital Select ◆ American Hospital Directory
◆ U.S. News Online ◆ Other Sites

Preplanning is key—whether you are choosing a doctor, making long-term fitness and nutrition goals, or deciding which hospital is right for you. What better way to begin making this decision than from the comfort of your home computer? Find listings of hospitals in your area, see data on the type and quality of care and services offered, and find out what others have to say.

Hospital Select

http://www.hospitalselect.com

 This division of Medical-Net has compiled detailed information on over 7,000 hospitals in the United States.

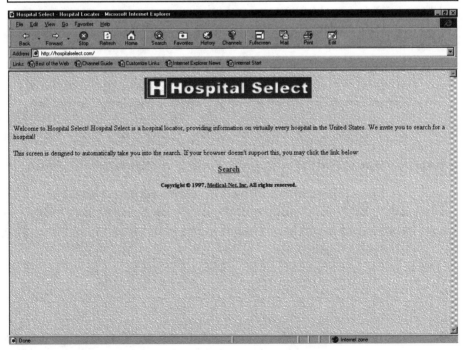

158

- This information-filled site allows you to search for a specific hospital by typing any part of the hospital name and the state where it is located. You also have the option of searching for a listing of hospitals in your city, county, or state.

- Select a hospital from the results list to see information such as phone numbers, address, number of beds, accreditation, admissions and emergency room admissions policies, services offered, and much more.

- If you have trouble searching the Hospital Select database, click the Search Tips button at the bottom of any page within the site.

- In addition to the hospital search, there are links to the American Medical Association, Physician Select, and Health Insight Home Web sites.

American Hospital Directory

http://www.ahd.com

This straightforward site, with information gathered from Medicare claims' data and other public files, is one of the best on the Web for hospital comparison shopping.

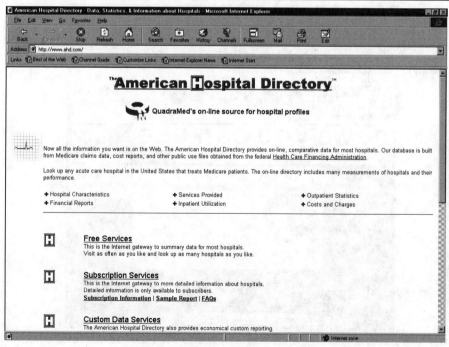

- This site's main goal is to give the public useful information so that they can effectively evaluate and compare hundreds of hospitals across the country. Begin by choosing the *Free Services* link on the home page. This is the "Internet gateway to summary data for most hospitals."

- Once you have searched for and found a hospital, you can scroll down the page for a list of services provided, as well as statistical information regarding staffing, ranking of services, average length of stay for Medicare patients, average charges for these stays, and more.

- Click the *Looking for Custom Data?* link on the home page to find out more about receiving custom reports, databases, and mailing lists for thousands of hospitals and hospital professionals.

U.S. News Online

**http://www.usnews.com/usnews/nycu/health/
hosptl/tophosp.htm**

 The Health area of this site has a searchable database of the 132 top-rated hospitals in the United States—according to a1998 *U.S. News & World Report* study of 6,400 hospitals.

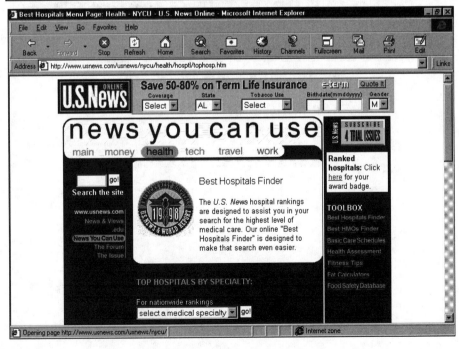

- This fabulous site allows you to conduct a hospital search nationwide, by specialty, state, and/or region. Once a search is completed and facilities are listed, each hospital is ranked and, when available, a link to its Web site is provided.

- The best feature of the *U.S. News* site is that it takes into account the fact that different hospitals excel in different areas of medicine. The hospital that may be best for treating cancer might not be the place for a heart bypass operation. The rankings listed, therefore, are based on medical specialty as well as geographic location.

- The site provides explanations of the methods used to select the best hospitals, as well as links to a glossary defining the medical terms and the types of services discussed. Also featured is an honor roll of the sixteen "top of the top" hospitals, chosen by *U.S News* using even more stringent criteria.

Other Sites

Virtual Hospital
http://vh.radiology.uiowa.edu

- This site is housed at the University of Iowa, and although many areas require a password to gain access, you can find a great deal of valuable medical information by simply clicking *For Patients* on the Virtual Hospital or Virtual Children's Hospital home page.

Health Scope
http://www.healthscope.org/hospital

- The Hospitals area of this site, especially the "Hospital Quality Checklist," outlines criteria and provides commonsense tips to help you home in on the right hospital.

Pedinfo
http://www.uab.edu/pedinfo

- This no-frills site is all about children's health care. From the comprehensive listing, select a site under the *Institutions* heading to see a list of children's hospitals, health care facilities, and advocacy organizations in the United States and around the world.

Mental Health

◆ **National Institute of Mental Health**
◆ **Mental Health Net** ◆ **Internet Mental Health**
◆ **Other Sites**

Although ten percent of all Americans suffer from some form of mental illness—from severe disorders to more manageable conditions—research is proving that many of these illnesses are diagnosable, treatable, and in many cases preventable. Numerous professional organizations, educational institutions, and mental health affiliates have established a presence on the Internet for the sole purpose of providing information, resources, and peace of mind for those who need help, their family, friends, and doctors.

National Institute of Mental Health

http://www.nimh.nih.gov

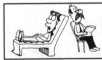 For the best mental health resources available online, visit the National Institutes of Health's NIMH site.

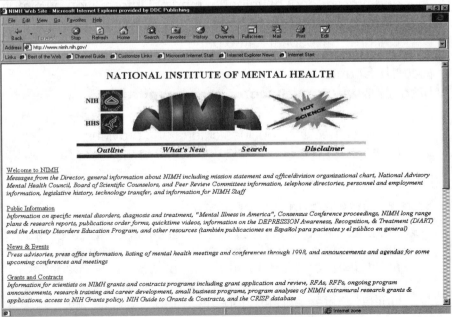

- This well-organized site is an excellent place to start your online search for mental health resources. For a quick peek at everything that's available, click the *Outline* link on the home page. You'll find resources for everything from specific mental disorders to programs and research reports.

- For information on various mental illnesses, click the *Public Information* link for a list of journal articles on diagnoses, treatments, research, and education programs. Or, click the *Hot Science* link to get detailed descriptions of common mental disorders and toll-free numbers you can call for free publications.

- To learn more about the latest scientific discoveries, click the *News & Events* link. Here you'll find press releases and news about upcoming mental health conferences and events.

Mental Health Net

http://www.cmhc.com

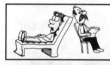
Whatever your questions about mental health may be, you can find answers at this comprehensive site that lists over 8,500 online resources.

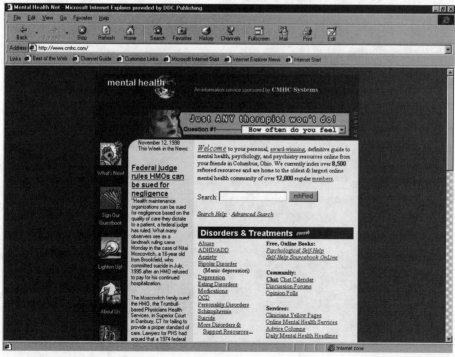

- This is an excellent site with a friendly tone, offering thousands of resources on mental disorders and treatments, online publications, community links, services, professional links, managed care information, news articles, humor, and more.

- Click the *Help* icon on the home page for a simple table of contents followed by detailed descriptions of news groups, Web resources, mailing lists, discussion groups, medical journals, and professional organizations.

- Mental Health Net has more than 12,000 members, placing it among the largest mental health communities online. You can participate in online chats, discussions, forums, opinion polls, and check the calendar of events to find out more about specific topics of interest.

Internet Mental Health

http://www.mentalhealth.com

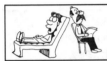
This award-winning Canadian site is a virtual encyclopedia of mental health resources on the World Wide Web.

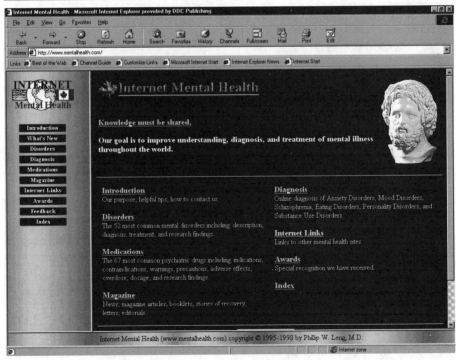

- Designed for mental health professionals, patients, friends and family members, support groups, students, and everyone who wants to learn more about mental health, this site has an abundance of information on mental disorders, treatments, medications, and research.

- The Magazine section contains professional articles, medical news, editorials, letters, and booklets, as well as numerous stories of recovery for uplifting reading.

- This site has a mammoth amount of readable, understandable information. If you are seeking a specific topic, use the index feature for quick access to hundreds upon hundreds of links. Even the number of Internet links to other mental health sites is staggering.

Other Sites

Psych Central™
http://psychcentral.com

- This site bills itself as "your personalized one-stop index for psychology." In addition to the Web resources and mental health information from other sites, Psych Central offers book reviews on relevant literature, live interactive chats, a suicide helpline, newsgroups, and mailing list information.

American Academy of Child & Adolescent Psychiatry
http://www.aacap.org

- This public service site is geared toward AACAP members, parents, and families who wish to learn more about child and adolescent psychiatry, research, managed care information, support, and more.

American Schools of Professional Psychology Learning Resources
http://www.aspp.edu/links_psych.html

- The Learning Resources page of this university Web site is a good source for links to Web sites on psychology, counseling, government resources, libraries, and health services. All listed links have been reviewed by the ASPP for quality and content.

MENTAL HEALTH

Nutrition & Fitness

◆ The American Dietetic Association ◆ PHYS
◆ Shape Up America ◆ Other Sites

Exercise—even moderate exercise—and a healthy diet are necessary ingredients for feeling and looking your best. More importantly, staying in shape and watching what you eat will alleviate and prevent many ailments and diseases. Although you can find sites dedicated to nutrition and fitness that cover everything from extreme bodybuilding to the latest diet crazes, try to home in on those that offer sensible advice from reputable sources.

The American Dietetic Association

http://www.eatright.org

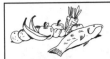 If you're looking for straightforward nutrition and general health advice for you and your family, ADA's site is a good place to start.

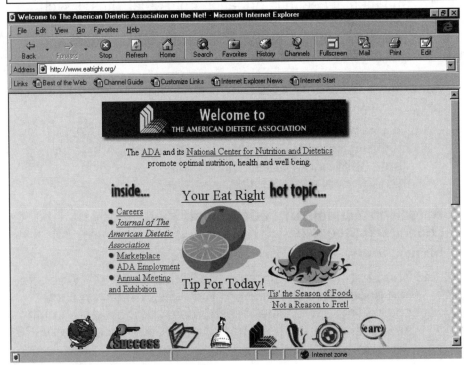

- Although a good part of the site is dedicated to professional dieticians, have no fear—there's a cornucopia of tips and additional resources available to everyone. Start with *Your Eat Right Tip of the Day!* for a quick piece of expert advice; then click the *Nutrition Resources* link and take your pick of categories, publications, and frequently updated features that are right for you.

- *Hot Topics* is definitely worth exploring. Find out about the Consumer Nutrition Hot Line (as well as how to contact a registered dietitian in your area) and click the link to *Nutrition Fact Sheets* (many include healthy recipes).

- Select *Search This Site* for immediate access to the ADA's resources regarding your particular point of interest.

PHYS

http://www.phys.com

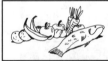 Geared toward nutrition and fitness for women, this site boasts expert advice from several national magazines.

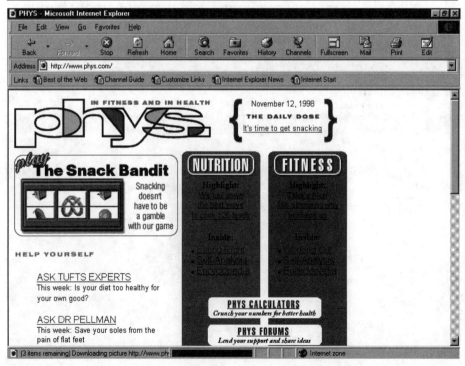

- PHYS features material from the publishers of six national magazines (including *Self* and *Women's Sports & Fitness*). Click one of the six magazine links at the bottom of the home page for the latest on fitness and nutrition. Or, perform a search to get relevant info from *all* the magazines—as well as from a host of other reputable sources.

- The PHYS site is conveniently divided into a "Fitness" section and a "Nutrition" section. Click the *Highlight* or *Inside* links of each for answers, tips, additional links, and more. (The tabs at the bottom of the home page also give you access to the two sections.)

- Appropriately enough, the layout of the site is very magazine-like, with fresh graphics, tie-ins to commercial products, and, of course, the magazine links themselves. But don't be fooled—for all its gloss, this site is filled with good, solid advice and practical information.

Shape Up America!

http://www.shapeup.org

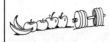 Founded by Dr. C. Everett Koop, Shape Up America! promotes weight management through healthy exercise and dietary habits.

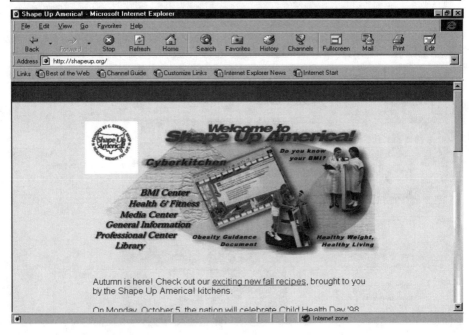

- Trying to shed a few pounds—for good? This site might be right for you. Click the *General Information* link, then choose *Our Mission* to get an idea of what Shape Up America! is all about.

- Even if losing weight is not your immediate health goal, this site is a good place to explore. If you're starting any sort of exercise program, click the *Health & Fitness* link to assess your fitness level. Then, for some good advice about eating right, check out the recipes offered on the site or enter the *Cyberkitchen*.

- Just what *is* "BMI"? It stands for "Body Mass Index." Click the *BMI Center* link and calculate your BMI. It's simple, and it's information you'll need as you plan your fitness and nutrition strategy.

Other Sites

Ask Dr. Weil
http://www.askdrweil.com

- Dr. Andrew Weil, M.D., the best-selling author of *Spontaneous Healing* and *8 Weeks to Optimum Health,* answers health and nutrition questions posted by visitors to the site. (See *General Medical Resources* for a more detailed look at the site.)

dietsite
http://www.dietsite.com

- Not only for dieters, this attractive site was created by a registered dietitian, who provides encyclopedia-style definitions of and commentary on a variety of nutrition and diet-related subjects. This site also offers links to other relevant Web sites, chat rooms, and a search feature. Great for anyone who wants to learn more about basic nutrition.

Fit-Net
http://www.fit-net.com

- Fit-Net is the first complete virtual fitness world. They are dedicated to bringing the "best and newest concepts" in health, exercise, and the nutrition to the user.

NUTRITION

169

Pediatrics

◆ **American Academy of Pediatrics**
◆ **KidsHealth at the AMA** ◆ **KidSource OnLine™**
◆ **Other Sites**

Our children are our future, so nurturing them and keeping them healthy are in everyone's best interest. Check out the following health care sites for parenting tips, advice from practicing professionals, and links to the most up-to-date books and articles on pediatric care.

American Academy of Pediatrics

http://www.aap.org

 AAP's site is a great source of information for both parents and pediatricians.

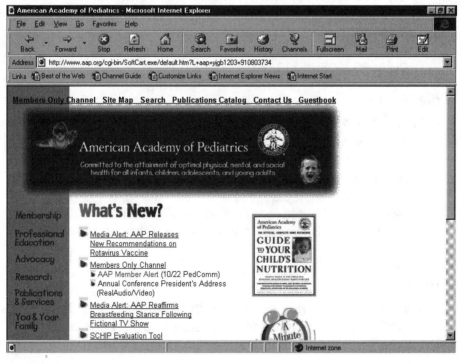

- Check out the *You & Your Family* link on the home page to find the latest services, programs, and resources available to you and your kids. Then visit the *Parent Resource Guide* area for a full list of "child care materials"—books, videos, and more, all geared toward answering any and all questions you have about your children's health.

- Medical professionals will find AAP membership information on the site. Benefits to members of AAP include up-to-date professional manuals and journals—important in providing your children's doctor with the most timely health information available.

KidsHealth at the AMA

http://www.ama-assn.org/KidsHealth

 This delightful site was developed by two trusted health authorities. Come here for medically reviewed information that's smartly categorized and easily accessible.

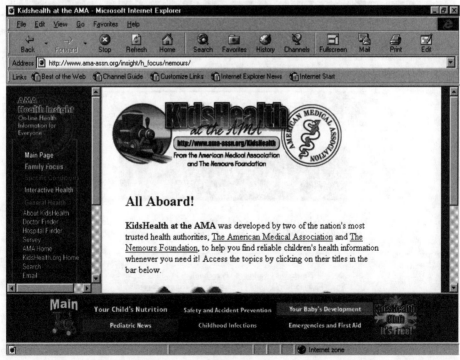

P
E
D
I
A
T
R
I
C
S

- Developed by the American Medical Association and the Nemours Foundation, this site features timely articles grouped into basic topic areas, such as *Your Child's Nutrition* and *Pediatric News*. All the material presented at this site has been created by a team of medical experts and professionals and reviewed by one or more children's health experts.

- Click one of the links at the bottom of every page to choose a topic area. You will then be treated to comprehensive articles and additional links tying in to your area of concern.

- The graphics throughout the site are fun, colorful, and kid-friendly. Browse with your kids, who will enjoy the pictures as much as you appreciate the expert information.

KidSource OnLine™

http://www.kidsource.com

 Developed by parents for parents (and their children, of course), this no-nonsense site is chock-full of valuable health and education resources.

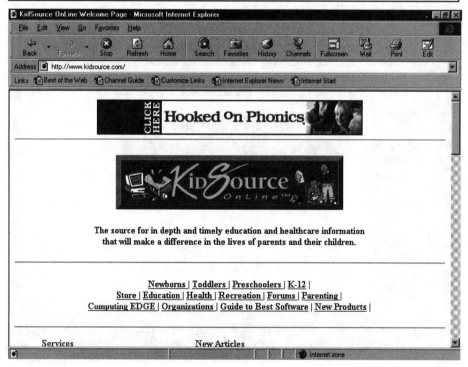

- Click the *About Us* link to see if this site is right for you. You might appreciate the fact that it is info-rich but light on graphics—this is intentional; KidSource wants you to be able to access their resources without having to wait for the pictures to load.

- KidSource emphasizes children's health and education—this is evident in their links to everything from reviews of new products to kid-friendly Web sites to articles about health care.

- Check out one of the KidSource OnLine Forums to share experiences with other parents—or browse the archives for previous discussions (e.g., *Car Seats, Children and Vitamins, Education and Kids,* and *Medical and Health Issues*).

Other Sites

The National Parenting Center
http://www.tnpc.com

- This award-winning site, brought to you by recognized authorities in the field of child-rearing, has helpful links to other parenting sites and health care resources.

Dr. Plain Talk™
http://www.drplaintalk.org

- This simple, straightforward site, sponsored by the Twin Cities' Childrens Hospitals and Clinics, offers pediatric health care information and answers to commonly asked questions.

Dr. Greene's HouseCalls
http://www.drgreene.com

- Dr. Greene, a practicing pediatrician dedicated to providing "pediatric wisdom for the information age," answers health care questions and leads you to additional materials of interest.

R$_X$ Corner

◆ RxList ◆ Healthtouch Online ◆ Other Sites

When faced with the thousands of over-the-counter remedies and prescriptions drugs used to cure or alleviate illness, there are times when you may want more information about a particular drug. For answers to questions about medications, their possible side effects, or clinical testing for FDA approval, consult any of the Web sites in this section.

RxList-The Internet Drug Index

http://www.rxlist.com

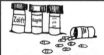 This well-trafficked, highly reputable site is one of the best resources for medication information on the Web.

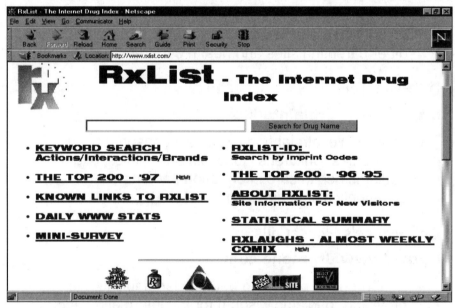

- The RxList database contains information on FDA-approved, or products close to approval, in the United States. There are over 4,000 products listed. However, the site notes that the information found on this site is only supplemental to information supplied by your physician.

- Search the database using the Keyword Search. From the results, you can find brand and generic names for medications, medical problems for which they might be used, side effects, and information on drug interaction.

- You can also find the Top 200 prescriptions written in the U.S. during the past three years. The drug's brand and generic names and manufacturer are listed. Clicking the generic name will direct you to information such as the average cost for a particular therapy, details for clinical studies, warnings, and recommendations for dosage and administration.

- There are hundreds of links to Web health sites listed under the *Known Links to RxList*.

Health*touch*®

http://www.healthtouch.com

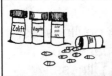 To learn about proper use, possible side effects, and general information on over 7,000 over-the-counter and prescription medications, consult the Heath*touch* database.

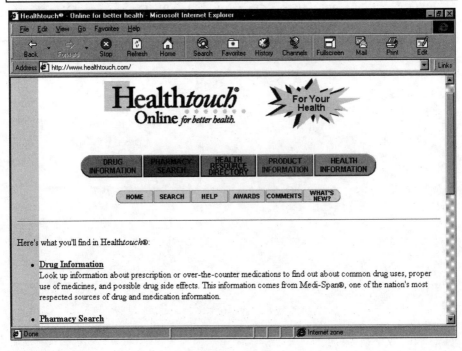

- The Health*touch* database draws its information from Medi-Span, reported to be one of the best sources for drug and medication information. Enter all, or even just part, of a medication's name to easily search this extensive database.

- Try clicking *Search* on the home page and enter the word *medications*. The Search Results display a range of helpful tips, such as what to ask your doctor about your prescription or how to organize a system of taking medications.

- Try clicking *Search* and entering the words *medicine terms*. The Search Results display the Health*touch* Dictionary of Medicine Terms, where you can find information about specific medical terms related to a medication.

- Health*touch* medical information can be accessed from automated machines located in pharmacies across the country. To find a pharmacy in your area with a Health*touch* machine, click the *Pharmacy Search* link from the home page and follow the onscreen directions.

- The site also holds a mine of other information on illnesses, symptoms, and treatments. Click *Health Information* to access the Table of Contents for information on illness, disease, and disorders. Go to the Health Resource Directory for a list of links to other health resource organizations.

Other Sites

New Medicines in Development

http://www.phrma.org/webdb/phrmawdb.html

- Learn about drugs that are still in the research and testing phase. You can search for information by disease, indication, or drug. The generic name for the new drug, the responsible pharmaceutical company name and location, and the status of current studies are included here.

MedWise, Inc

http://www.mailmedicine.com/

- MedWise claims to be able to fill any prescription for IV fluids, over-the-counter drugs, homeopathic products, and more. They offer competitive prices, including senior citizen discounts. Your order can be delivered by mail or courier within 72 hours.

PharmInfoNet

http://pharminfo.com/

- Visit this site for any kind of information on pharmaceuticals. It provides patient resources, including reports on clinical trials and patient newsgroups. Get answers to questions about different drugs and drug therapies from a wide-ranging list of topics.

R
x
C
O
R
N
E
R

Sleep Disorders

◆ SleepNet ◆ National Sleep Foundation
◆ The Sleep Medicine Home Page ◆ Other Sites

Is getting a good night's sleep an impossible dream? Then you may be one of 50 million Americans who suffers from a sleep disorder. The good news is you can rest assured that there are thousands of resources at your fingertips. In the blink of an eye, you'll be able to find detailed information on all kinds of sleep disorders, how they're treated, and where you can turn for support, advice, and medical care.

SleepNet

http://www.sleepnet.com

 The ultimate sleep site on the Internet, SleepNet has information, support, and links galore.

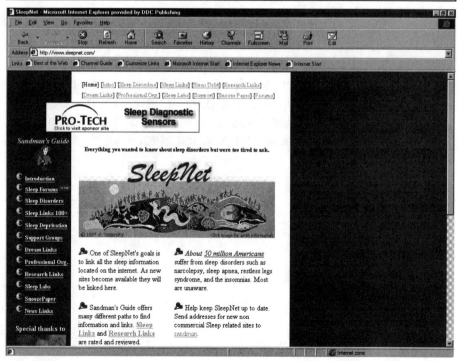

- This charming, artfully designed site provides the "Sandman's Guide" to sleep information online. SleepNet's goal is to be the clearinghouse of all sleep-related sites. If you're looking to learn more about sleep and sleep disorders, this is a great place to start.

- Click *Sleep Links* on the home page to get "owl" rated reviews and descriptions of sites specific to insomnia, narcolepsy, sleep apnea, sleepwalking, restless leg syndrome, infant and child sleep problems, sleep and aging, and others.

- Read telltale descriptions of various sleep disorders, and find out where you can turn for help. SleepNet has links to professional organizations, support groups, sleep forums, sleep labs, research centers, and related news stories.

National Sleep Foundation

http://www.sleepfoundation.org

 This nonprofit organization promotes increased awareness of all aspects of sleep, prevention of sleep-related disorders, and expanded research and public policy.

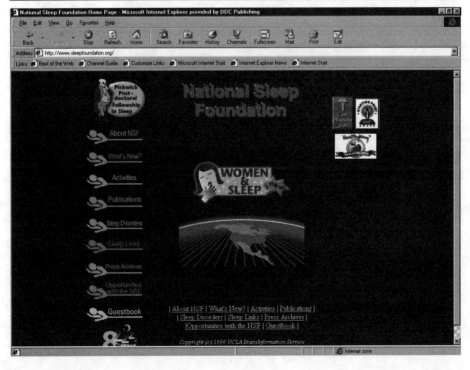

S
L
E
E
P

D
I
S
O
R
D
E
R
S

- This award-winning site is an excellent source for improving your awareness about the importance of sleep. The National Sleep Foundation has numerous online brochures about specific sleep disorders that describe symptoms and common treatments, and which offer facts, self-tests, and resources for medical advice or care.

- In addition to providing sleep links, press archives, e-zines, and other publications, the NSF encourages participation in various sleep-awareness campaigns and programs. You can sign a confidential registry to receive publications and be informed of events and activities.

The Sleep Medicine Home Page
http://www.users.cloud9.net/~thorpy

 This straightforward, but information-filled, site is one long page of links to sleep resources.

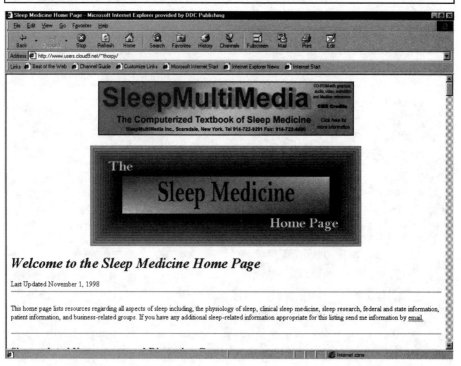

- The Sleep Medicine Home Page is a great source for sleep links to newsgroups, online forums, discussion groups, and FTP sites. In addition to sleep disorder links, you can find databases, medical journal sites, and sites related to dreams and psychology.

- Find extensive lists of national and international professional associations, organizations, businesses, and foundations. You can also read articles and reviews on medications and research studies.

- The Sleep Medicine Home Page has an extensive list of sleep disorder centers in the United States and all around the world. You can link to those facilities that have Web sites; otherwise, institute, city, and country information is provided.

Other Sites

American Sleep Disorders Association
http://www.asda.org

- The ASDA site provides excellent links for sleep disorder information and shows you where to find available educational material, patient support groups, organizations, and medical research centers.

Doctor's Guide® to Insomnia Information & Resources
http://www.pslgroup.com/insomnia.htm

- Can't sleep? Check out this site for links to the latest news in medical breakthroughs, support groups, and patient resources for insomnia-related disorders. You can request e-mail notification of new links and changes to the site.

The Sleep Well
http://www.stanford.edu/~dement

- Started by the director of the Stanford University Sleep Disorders Clinic and Laboratory, the Sleep Well is a great source for research news, views, treatment information, literature, health and medical links, and material on accredited sleep centers across the country.

SLEEP DISORDERS

Women's Health

Mothers, daughters, sisters, aunts, and grandmothers all have one thing in common: the female body. And this body goes through many changes over the years. Stay informed with what is going on with your body or find answers to health questions for women who are near and dear to you. Read up on women's health, issues, and research breakthroughs online.

OBGYN.net

http://www.obgyn.net/women/women.htm

 This site runs the gamut of information—everything from child rearing to menopause to finding a doctor and reading the latest in medical research.

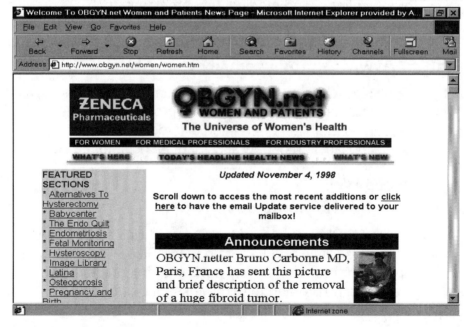

- Consider this site women's health central, with an incomparable number of links, support chat groups, featured articles, doctor directories, and more—all information pertaining to women's wellness.

- The best way to navigate this site is to scroll through the topics in the left column of the page and then click a link that interests you. The site is divided into eleven major headings, including Health Information, Interactive Tools (such as finding a doctor or looking up acronyms), and Organizations. In addition, the home page features articles.

- You can also sign up for a free direct e-mail service that will keep you informed of the latest developments at OBGYN.net. Subscribers receive brief updates (usually just a few paragraphs) once or twice a week.

Foundation for Osteoporosis Research and Education
http://www.fore.org

 Osteoporosis is a disease that affects over 25 million Americans. There are some simple dos and don'ts that can help you beat these odds. Check out this nonprofit, educational site for lots of information.

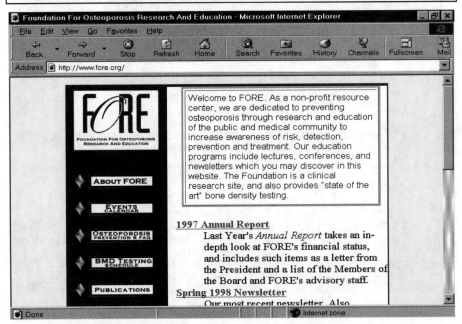

- The old adage, "an ounce of prevention is worth a pound of cure," could be this site's motto. FORE stresses education about osteoporosis as a means to avoid getting this debilitating disease.

- Though it's best to start preventative measures when you are young and your bones are developing, it is never too late to start good habits.

- This site provides an abundance of articles, information, FAQs (frequently asked questions), support for those with osteoporosis, and excellent health guidelines for those without.

Menopause Online

http://www.menopause-online.com

 This site is dedicated to providing women (and the men who love them) support, strength, and up-to-date information about menopause.

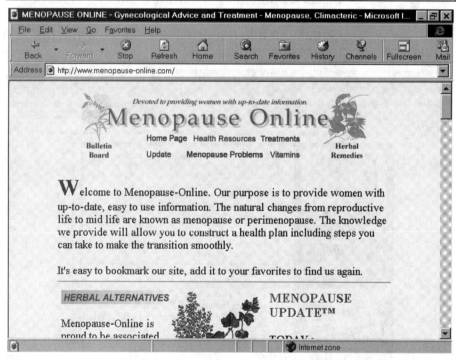

- This site focuses on integrative measures for dealing with the changes that a woman's body undergoes as she experiences menopause. This includes combining healthy diet and exercise with herbal remedies, vitamins, acupuncture, and homeopathy.

- Menopause online also features the latest scientific studies, health resources, and a bulletin board system where you can post questions or share your experiences, and more.

Other Sites

Welcome to BreastNet™
http://www.bci.org.au

- This site—sponsored by the NSW Breast Cancer Institute—is divided into three sections: BCI, which explains the goal of the Institute; Medical, which includes new studies, research, and date; and Public, the area of the site that includes general information, care options, and women's stories about their battle with breast cancer.

National Women's Health Resource Center
http://www.healthywomen.org

- This award-winning national clearinghouse is an excellent site for women's resources online. Find hundreds of links to subject-specific sites, family links, alternative medicine, aging, cervical cancer, fitness, and fertility, just to name a few.

Women's Health Directory
http://www.health-library.com/women/index.html

- This is a good place to start your search for links to specific women's health topics, including breast cancer, pregnancy, contraception, menopause, female sexuality, PMS, mental health, and more.

185

Medical Appendix

This section provides resources for more specialized medical and health topics not covered in previous topics. The sites under each heading are good launch pads for further research because of the number of Web links they provide.

AIDS/HIV Resources

AIDS Resources List

http://www.teleport.com/~celinec/aids.shtml

- This site contains hundreds of links to national, regional, and international sites on the subject of AIDS/HIV. Among these expert sources, you can read the latest findings about AIDS/HIV transmission, treatment and prevention, and how this disease affects children and adults alike. You'll also find a collection of support-group Web sites (such as the Safer Sex Page and AIDS NOW! Project for Teens), human interest stories, international HIV magazines, medical sites for caregivers, and much more.

Doctor's Guide to AIDS Information & Resources

http://www.pslgroup.com/AIDS.htm

- Come to this site for hundreds of articles on new treatments, medical findings, and drug therapies. This site is also a useful source for links to other Web sites relevant to AIDS education, research, and support. In addition, you can find discussion forums, newsgroups, and online chat groups.

Alcoholism

Alcoholics Anonymous
http://www.alcoholics-anonymous.org

- According to Alcoholics Anonymous, you are the only one who can decide whether or not you have an addiction to alcohol. If you suspect that you may have a problem, read answers to questions about alcoholism in the area called A Newcomer Asks or take the Is A.A. for You? quiz. Search the A.A. database to find a meeting in your area. The information on this site is available in English, Spanish, and French.

Alcoholism.Net
http://www.alcoholism.net

- Alcoholism.Net is a comprehensive, one-stop site on all things concerning alcoholism. Find links to support newsgroups and chat rooms, general information about alcohol abuse and treatments, recovery resources, and more.

Alzheimer's Disease

Alzheimers.com
http://www.alzheimers.com

- This highly acclaimed site offers daily articles written on different facets of Alzheimer's, a searchable database of over 3,800 professional biomedical journals, and a pen-pal support community bulletin board. You'll also find terrific information on how to be an effective caregiver to an afflicted loved one or friend.

The Alzheimer's Association
http://www.alz.org

- The Alzheimer's Association offers information on the most recent advances in the treatment of the disease, in addition to the latest news about possible cures. This site has helpful support for people with Alzheimer's and their caregivers as well as resources that can help you gain a better understanding of this affliction.

Clinical Trials and Medical Breakthroughs

Medical Breakthroughs

http://www.ivanhoe.com

- This site, brought to you by Ivanhoe Broadcast News, posts the latest reports on medical breakthroughs. Read articles, see videos, and catch daily news flashes on today's medical breakthroughs and tomorrow's cures.

Center Watch: Clinical Trials Listing Service

http://www.centerwatch.com

- Find a listing of new drug therapies that have been FDA-approved in the past three years. You'll also find extensive information on clinical trials, including material for those who may be interested in participating. This site is also a good source for listings of over 100 health associations.

Eating Disorders

The American Anorexia/Bulimia Association, Inc

http://members.aol.com/amanbu

- Did you know that over five million Americans suffer from eating disorders? If you would like to learn more about anorexia, bulimia, binge-eating disorder, and how to detect early warning signs, consult this site. This is an excellent place to learn about symptoms and possible cures for those who are afflicted. If you or someone you know is seeking help, click *information for those who suffer from eating disorders* to find and evaluate potential therapists.

The Center for Eating Disorders

http://www.eating-disorders.com

- In addition to articles that shed light on different eating disorders and their possible causes, this site offers extensive support channels. Join an online discussion and ask questions of or read answers from resident experts. This site's goal is to teach others how to cope and offer solutions on how to get back on the road to healthy living.

Lyme Disease

Lyme Disease Information Resource

http://www.x-l.net/Lyme

- Visit this site for a general overview of Lyme disease and other tick-borne diseases. You'll find extensive scientific information about medical research, links to Web resources that describe the symptoms and available treatment, and numerous support group listings. Be sure to access the picture gallery's photos of ticks and rashes to increase your awareness of potential warning signs.

American Lyme Disease Foundation, Inc.

http://www.aldf.com

- The Centers for Disease Control and Prevention have reviewed and approved all the information posted at this site. Learn more about Lyme disease and other tick-borne infections, order inexpensive pamphlets, and read late-breaking news related to the treatment and prevention of Lyme disease.

Outreach and Support Groups

Health Information Resources

http://nhic-nt.health.org/scripts/tollfree.cfm

- If you have specific questions or just want to talk to someone, check out this site for toll-free numbers to hundreds of health organizations that provide support and medical information.

Clinical Trials.com

http://www.clinicaltrials.com

- Although this site's primary focus is clinical trials studies and the latest information on newly approved drug therapies, their Support Services area has an extensive database. To find community support near you, click the *Support Services* link and choose from over thirty medical topics, including HIV/AIDS, neurology, and drug treatments.

Sexually Transmitted Diseases

Unspeakable: The Naked Truth About STDs

http://www.unspeakable.com/std-index.html

- If you want to know "the naked truth" about sexually transmitted diseases, this is the place to visit. The language is frank and the approach to this subject is no-nonsense. Learn the facts about STDs, locate a clinic in your area for treatment, find answers to frequently asked questions, and get sage advice on how to discuss STDs with your partner.

American Social Health Association

http://sunsite.unc.edu/ASHA

- The American Social Health Association's mission is to "stop sexually transmitted diseases (STDs) and their harmful consequences to individuals, families, and communities." To this end, they provide a variety of educational resources, numerous links to STD hotlines, a glossary of relevant terms, and a listing of support groups in your area.

Smoking

Blair's Quitting Smoking Resources

http://www.chriscor.com

- So you have finally made the decision to stop smoking. The question now is how to conquer your addiction to nicotine. Before you reach for that next cigarette, read how others are doing it by going to Blair's Quitting Smoking Discussion Board or by joining Blair's Quit Smoking Discussion Group. You'll also find over sixty links to excellent Web sites, each offering medical facts and suggestions on healthy ways to help you quit.

190

The Ashtray: Smoking and Tobacco Abuse
http://www.bu.edu/cohis/smoking/smoke.htm

- This no-frills site offers just the facts about cigarette smoking, including why people smoke and how it harms the body. The Ashtray also offers tips on how to stop. Although the treatments discussed here are brief, this site is a good launching point for learning more about smoking cessation techniques and treatments. Find out about new medications on the market, behavioral modification, and alternative techniques such as aversion therapy.

Substance Abuse

Drug-Free Resource Net
http://www.drugfreeamerica.org

- The Partnership for a Drug-Free America provides answers to frequently asked questions about drugs. See pictures of what specific drugs look like and learn more about their effects on the body. Partnership for a Drug-Free America guarantees that all the information presented on the site is up-to-date and accurate. Parents can find drug education information, support organizations, and recommended Web resources.

Go Ask Alice!
http://www.goaskalice.columbia.edu

- "Alice" is a team of health educators and health care providers at Columbia University in New York City and around the world. According to the site, readers in sixty countries consult Alice 2.5 million times a month on any number of drug-related topics. Read answers from health care professionals to thousands of letters submitted by visitors to the site. Go Ask Alice! covers many drugs not found on other drug-related Web sites including "club" drugs such as Ketamine ("Special K"), MDMA ("X" or "Ecstasy"), and GHB ("Liquid Ecstasy"). Alice guarantees that all posted information and advice are researched for quality and accuracy.

Transplants and Organ Donorship

TransWeb

http://www.transweb.org

- TransWeb answers common questions about transplants and organ donation. Their goal is to dispel myths and misunderstandings by providing facts about the transplantation process, and include stories from those who have received and donated organs and tissue.

RenalNet

http://www.renalnet.org

- RenalNet is the recipient of numerous awards for the outstanding Web resources the site offers. Kidney diseases affect millions of people in the United States. For more information on the causes of and treatments for these debilitating ailments, visit RenalNet.

Index

O

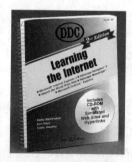
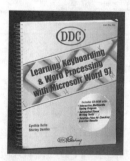
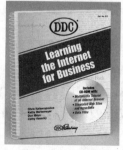
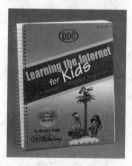

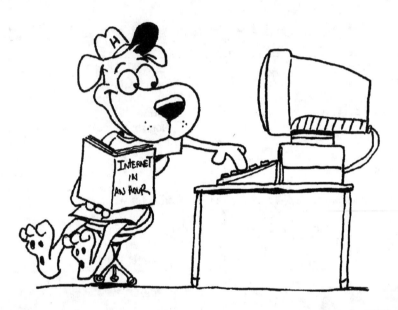